"CHALLENGES ARE NOT A SIGN OF FAILURE,
BUT AN OPPORTUNITY FOR DEVELOPMENT"

CONTENTS

INSIDE

10 MARCH 2022
SELECTED ARTICLES

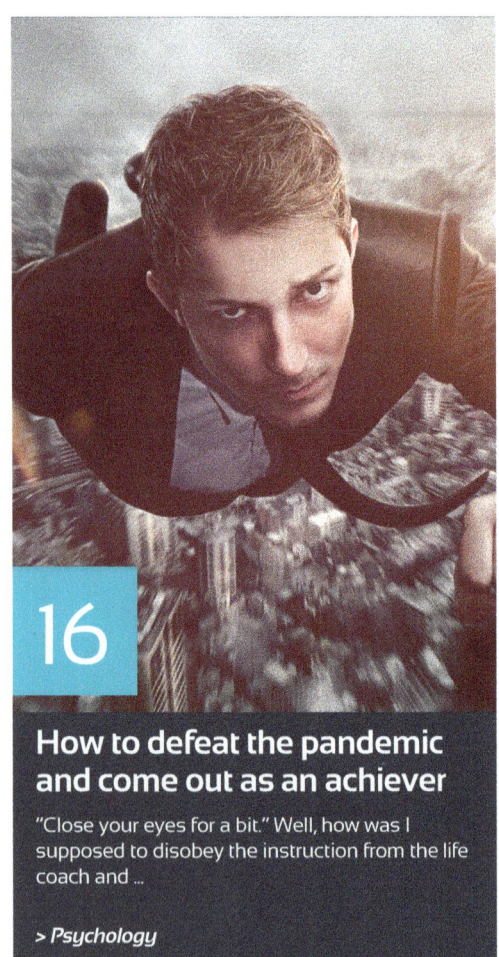

16

How to defeat the pandemic and come out as an achiever

"Close your eyes for a bit." Well, how was I supposed to disobey the instruction from the life coach and ...

> Psychology

04

Neuro-Linguistic Programming (NLP)
A brief overview

Neuro-Linguistic Programming (NLP) is a psychological approach that learns, analyses, and applies the strategies by reframing the way we think and see the world to achieve personal goals.

> Psychology

04

Hypnotherapy Specializations, Techniques & Tools

Hypnosis is an altered and yet natural state of the conscious mind that can be naturally used for therapeutic purposes with the option to amend unwanted habits and behaviours.

> Hypnotherapy

20

The efficiency and limitations of online hypnotherapy

The effectiveness of online hypnotherapy is currently not quite clear, therefore in 2020 a survey collecting statistical data about common cases performed online was conducted and the collected data may serve for further exploration.

> Hypnotherapy

26

Why Research of Clinical Hypnotherapy Must Flourish

"Hypnotherapy must be doing something right because it keeps coming back into the medical field. My message to the drug companies is if you invest, we shall do the research on hypnotherapy for you, and eventually, it will bring the profit to you,"...

> Hypnotherapy

35

Is there a life after the Pandemic?

A positive afternoon with Wayne Farrell

> Interviews

Welcome

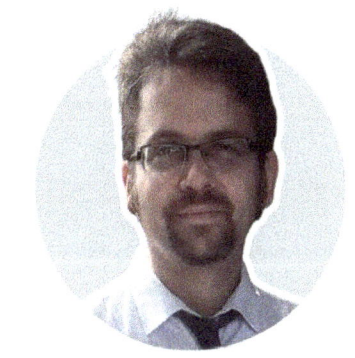

Although the pandemic seems to be nearly over, you can find articles in this magazine that were written during the most challenging times and deal with this topic. Perhaps it is now more obvious that a postpandemic state will have its consequences not only on mental health, and in such times it is more than useful to work with professionals, for instance a hypnotherapist.

Challenges are not a sign of failure, but an opportunity for development, so even though they may be unpleasant they will ultimately show how we develop. We can become stronger, more confident, and happier. Hypnotherapy can provide an insight into how far we have come and dysfunctional beliefs can easily be changed.

This issue contains articles for professionals and for those looking for help or inspiration. Not all articles have been added to the contents. On page five you can find a brief overview of neurolinguistic programming. Page eight has an article about how antidepressants work. Page eleven is about transcranial direct current stimulation. On page twelve is a review of specializations, techniques, and tools in hypnotherapy. Page seventeen has inspiring guidelines from Mike Pegg about how to defeat the pandemic and come out as an achiever. On page twenty is a paper about the efficiency and limitations of online hypnotherapy. Page twenty-four is a hypothesis about the inherited role of the child formed by dominance within the family. Page twenty-seven brings an inspiring interview with Mr. Peter Mabbutt about why research of clinical hypnotherapy must flourish. On page thirty you can find the directory of hypnotherapy. On page thirty-two is an interview with an educator of clinical hypnotherapy, Hansruedi Wipf. And finally, page thirty-five brings an inspiring interview with Wayne Farrell about whether there is life after the pandemic.

I believe that our magazine will find its place among your favourite titles. On behalf of the editorial team I wish you pleasant reading.

> *Jakub Tencl, Ph.D. - Editor in Chief*

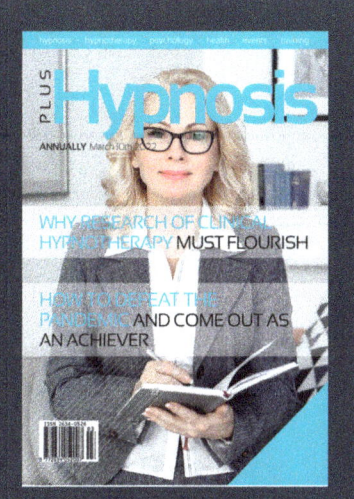

Editor in chief and publisher: Jakub Tencl, Ph.D. T. 08431223206 (Calls to this number are charged at 5p/min plus your network access charge) E. info@hypnosis.plus | **Editor:** Leiden Delpassen E. editor@hypnosis.plus | **Publisher's postal address:** Unit 16685, PO Box 6945, London, W1A 6US | **Contact for an advertisement:** adverts@hypnosis.plus | **Contact for subscriptions:** 07537171272 E. subscription@hypnosis.plus | The magazine is published annually and printed at Amazon.com, Inc. | Published on March 10th 2022 | **Source of unsigned photos:** Dreamstime.com | Authors of unsigned photos: Siarhei Yurchanka, Viktoriia Hnatiuk, Pressmaster, Fizkes, Andrey Popov, Nikki Zalewski, Anatoliygleb | **Cover Photo:** dreamstime.com | **Price:** £7 ($9) | Unsolicited articles will not be returned. | The editorial team reserves the right to shorten or edit texts. | The published texts may not have to express the opinions and attitudes of the editorial team and the publisher. | ISSN 2634-0526

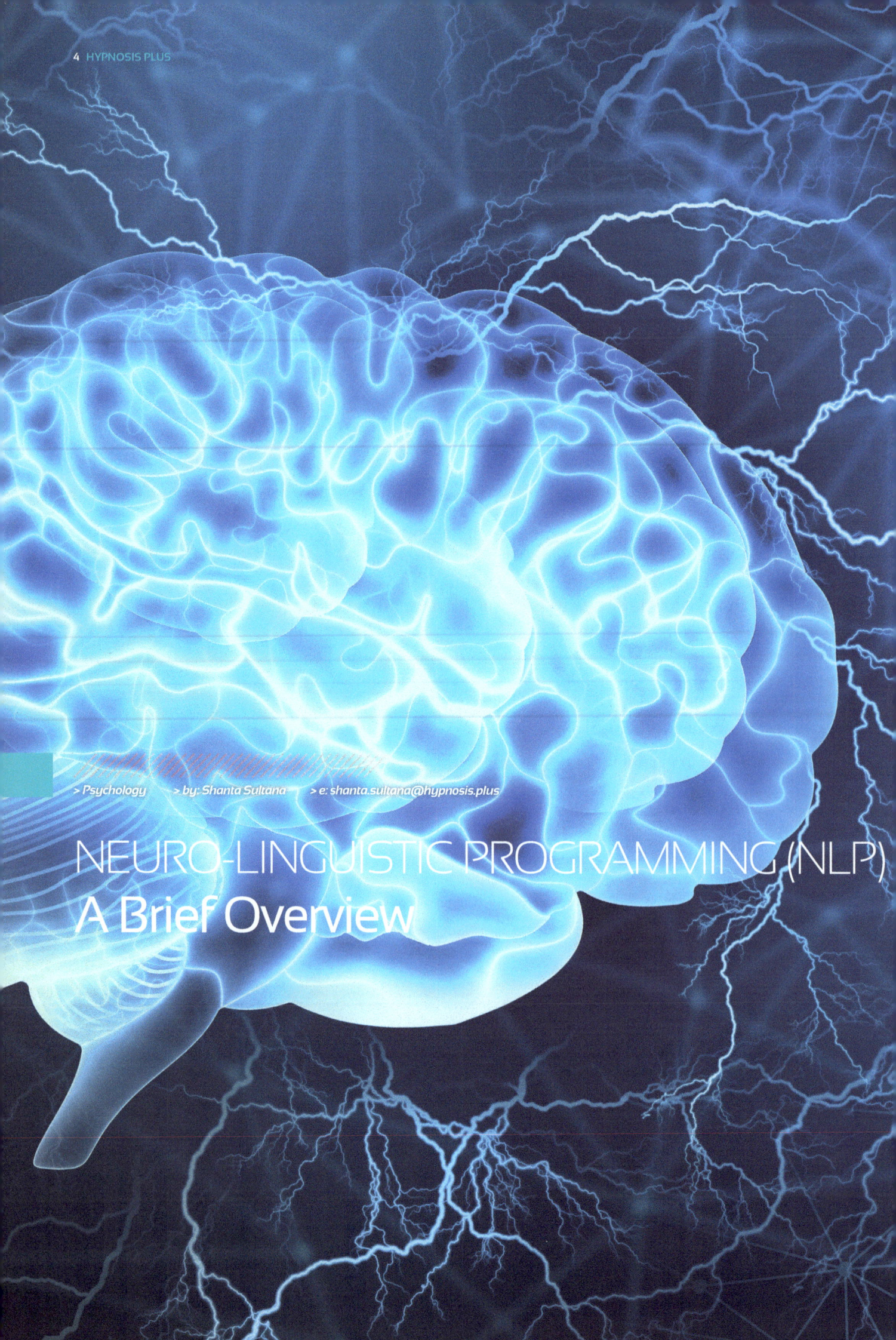

> Psychology   > by: Shanta Sultana   > e: shanta.sultana@hypnosis.plus

NEURO-LINGUISTIC PROGRAMMING (NLP)
A Brief Overview

PSYCHOLOGY

Neuro-Linguistic Programming (NLP)
A Brief Overview

Neuro-Linguistic Programming (NLP) is a psychological approach that learns, analyses, and applies the strategies by reframing the way we think and see the world to achieve personal goals. This article will explore what NLP is and know about its creators, understand the basic theory, if it is scientifically proven, and its effects on the brain.

It can be stated that the belief of NLP advocates is all human actions are positive; if something fails, it is neither a good or bad experience but is useful information that can be used to achieve the goals (Good Therapy).

There are numerous interviews of Richard Bandler, the co-creator of NLP, talking about reframing the way we think to see all experiences as useful information or as an opportunity. Bandler states that he had been studying successful people to understand how they can accomplish targets with the power of positive thinking. That people continuously think or see things from a negative angle and lose the opportunity to find a positive solution.

Such as:

Thought one: "If I am made redundant from my job, I shall have a difficult future, and it is out of my control."

Thought two "If I am made redundant, this is an opportunity to do something I always wanted to do, and I can make a new start."

With thought one, a person may use the coach and stop focusing on what might go wrong and develop fear. The fear may withhold the subject from thinking creatively about what to do to turn this adverse situation into a good one.

With thought two, a person may start focusing on what can be done next. The thinking process may enable the subject to be active and reach out to people and start new tasks.

Another example of reframing the thinking process is when we think we are thinking positively, but in reality, we embed fear and anxiety in the subconscious. For example, "Please don't miss this interview;" by saying such things, we send a message to ourselves that we may mess this up. Here, NLP practitioners say that every negative thought process has a positive intention. If we ask ourselves what it is that we want and work on it from there, we can then work on the positive intention instead of that negative thought. So if the subject asks what is desired from the interview, the subject then can ask what can be done to give the best performance possible. Therefore, the subject will do everything that needs to be done, such as research, demonstrative practice, and send the message to self that they have completed all the tasks to be prepared for the interview; hence, it will be a positive experience. That can help the subject release fear and anxiety, so the performance would be better.

It is possible to think that life is full of negative events. But the belief is that these negative events have positive intentions, so the question can be asked what is it we want and how can we use these negative events to achieve our goals. Therefore, every event can be seen as an opportunity.

It can be stated that the above theory is about changing the way people think. It does not tell us if NLP is affecting the brain. Therefore, despite NLP being immensely successful worldwide, the scientific communities still haven't accepted NLP as a rational method.

Let's look at the brief history of NLP:

An American scientist and mathematician Richard Bandler and a linguist John Grinder became interested in making effective changes in people's lives during the 1970s and observed successful but unorthodox therapists throughout the United States. They studied these therapists were using a certain pattern of a verbal and non-verbal communication system which had profound positive effects, and they monitored that although superficially the therapists used individual models, there were some common denominators in the usage of language patterns in the subconscious level. The scientists refined and tested these patterns on a large number of volunteers. After applying the newly invented approach, there was a dramatic shift in the volunteers' "approach to life" within a short period. Again, Bandler talks about how people were thinking in the 60s and 70s in a number of interviews on social networks where he states that there was a general understanding that "Changes takes time." The volunteers' new approach to life stood against this traditional concept. The new methodology was named Neuro-Linguistic Programming. Addressing three driving forces of human actions and interactions: Neurology, Communication, and Behaviour. Bandler declared that he came up with the name Neuro-Linguistic Programming on a whim because it sounded good. Therefore, the word Neuro can be misleading as it suggests that it has a neurological approach. Nevertheless, Many NLP practitioners say that NLP changes the way the brain works, but this is not accepted by the scientific communities to this date.

Therefore, it is vital that we continue to explore if NLP techniques make any neurological changes.

According to some practitioners' explanation, the way a human communicates with self and with others (linguistic, verbal, body language, or sign language) affects the nervous system (Neuro), which then sets up a pattern of behavior (Programming); therefore, these ways of communication can be amended or altered; effective internal processing can result in a rewarding life.

There has not been any scientific research to prove the above yet. There are many different methods practiced by NLP practitioners worldwide, and there is no set method or explanation. According to critics, the above explanation is generalizing, and the evidence found is anecdotal. Therefore, this is not a scientific explanation.

Bandler and Grinder studied psychologists Fritz Perls, Virginia Satir, and Milton Erickson; Their two most influential models are The Meta Model based on Satir and Perls and the renowned Milton Model based on Erickson.

Bandler and Grinder published a book based on the study in 1975, and NLP was developed at the University of California, Santa Cruz. They successfully marketed it, and it has been learned and experienced by over 200,000 people in the USA (Dr. Kotera, Y) and millions worldwide since the 1980s (Good Therapy; William, C; 2012). It has been argued that Bandler and Grinder were focused on creating a profitable theory and knew how to sell it to the world. The fact that so many people have bought the idea makes it even more believable. Cynics say that Brandler and Grinder were students around the time; they came up with the idea, and they advertised NLP as a powerful persuasion technology. Hence, it became a highly profitable business; the main intention was to generate revenue from this idea (Hutton;2017).

Dr. Yasuhiro Kotera, the Academic Lead in Counselling, Psychotherapy, and Psychology at the University of Derby, explains that the reason NLP research is scientifically underdeveloped is that there is no established systematic approach or explanations. Each practitioner has a creative tool. However, there are no set criteria for NLP qualification, and the titles for study modules are inconsistent around the globe. There is no supervision process for continuous personal development or regulations to maintain an international standard of teaching, practicing, and learning. Dr. Kotera says that NLP is a useful tool in psychotherapy and has clinical application. NLP offers a quicker intervention and explains, "NLP is an approach to communication and personal development that focuses on how individuals organize their thinking, feelings, and language.

It has been identified a number of explanations available for NLP. As an example, a brief definition of NLP by practitioners:

PSYCHOLOGY

Neuro: Individuals experience reality differently through the five senses. Neuro is about the neurological system, based on the idea that we experience the world through our senses and translate sensory information into our thought processes in both conscious and unconscious levels. These thought processes activate the neurological system, and this affects our psychology, emotions, and behavior.

Linguistic (also non-verbal): This is how individuals use language to make sense of the world, capture and conceptualize experiences, and communicate with others based on these experiences. How the individual uses the words influences the experience. These experiences go through five senses visual (images), auditory (sounds), kinaesthetic (touch and internal feelings), gustatory (tastes), and olfactory (smells) senses. The experience we gather via the five senses is expressed via words, signs, and body language.

Programming: The sensory experiences and internal processing represent a pattern with a specific outcome and behavior pattern affecting the general make-up of the individual life. An individual has personal programming consisting of internal processing of gathered experiences and then forming internal strategies to communicate with the world. This helps to make decisions, evaluate experiences, approaches to learning, solve problems, and get outcomes. (William, C; P: 14-15; 2012)

It can be stated that there is a number of NLP strategies around the world because each internal strategies are unique and needs to be understood by the NLP coach. There are claims that NLP methodology is based on cognitive psychology. Richard Bandler defines NLP as "NLP is an attitude which is an insatiable curiosity about human beings with a methodology that leaves behind it a trail of techniques. "

John Grinder explains, "The strategies, tools, and techniques of NLP represent an opportunity unlike any other for the exploration of human functioning, or more precisely, that rare and valuable subset of human functioning known as genius. "

The above explanations tell that NLP is a powerful tool with a series of methods and techniques. However, it does not mean it is based on neuroscience.

NLP practitioners focus on:

Purpose and Spirituality: Thank to step by step methodology, teaches a sincere desire to live a spiritual life helping the client make positive changes in behaviors, communication, and the ability to solve problems; hence, some practitioners claim that the highest level of changes happens here.

Identity: What are the roles in one's life?

Beliefs and Values: What matters to the person?

Capabilities & Skills: Individual Capacity.

Behaviors: Specific actions

Environment: The lowest level of change happen here (Good Therapy)

NLP has been applied in a variety of professional grounds in the UK and USA. DWP and independent businesses have hired NLP coaches for people to work productively in job searches and in their designated roles. The UK Council of Psychotherapy accepted NLP in 1990. The NHS embedded NLP training in 2006-2009 and the UK Teachers Training sector trained tutors in NLP in 2003-2016 (Dr. Kotera, Y)

The debate

Despite its success, NLP is still not acknowledged as mainstream psychology, and limited research is available. The British Psychological Society (BPS) does not acknowledge it. It is argued that NLP is simple to learn yet a very powerful tool sold as a brand. Therefore, anyone with or without a specific qualification in psychology and neuroscience can become an NLP practitioner. It is a great business opportunity for charismatic individuals. That Bandler & Grinder didn't create a new tool, and the title NLP is meaningless but designed to influence people to think it is a scientifically proven method. The ideas are copied from previous practitioners; Richard Bandler was a student at the University of California, and John Grinder was the Assistant Professor of Linguistics at the time they came up with the theories of NLP. Bandler was asked to transcribe sessions by a therapist who wanted to write a book based on the recorded transcriptions. Bandler used these recorded therapy sessions and identified useful language patterns. He then took these patterns to the professor, and they studied how they worked, and this was when NLP was discovered. Copying recorded therapy sessions would be illegal today; however, there was no law in 1960-70, and people were interested in new things in this era. Therefore, it was a huge opportunity for Brandler and Grinder to market it as a teaching tool. Hence, it is argued that it is a method that was copied and mixed with few other things and had no scientific value. Branding is important to market an idea, and NLP is a catchy brand identity (Hutton; 2017).

Therefore, NLP is a collection of techniques that are used by people who naturally use them. Some people are naturally persuasive than others, so it does not help everyone. I.e., when, in 2015, the UK Department of Work and Pension sent the unemployed to NLP training for a positive approach in finding work, users reported that they were made to feel they were responsible for their disposition. It was compulsory to attend the NLP training; the jobseekers expressed that the courses suggested the reason they were unemployed and could not find employment in a set time was because of the way they were communicating, speaking, and seeing the world. That it was not the economic, political, social, and cultural reasons that were making the job sector hard to reach. It was down to them. If they changed their way of approaching the world and vision, they would find suitable employment. The jobseekers felt it was patronizing, and the DWP was detached from the reality (Benefit & Work Guides; 2015).

The British Medical Journal (BMJ), a subsidiary of BPS, condemned it (Benefits & Work Guides; 2015). It is argued that persuasive people such as politicians have always been using NLP without studying it as it is their natural state of character. NLP has a placebo effect because the trainers are persuasive in making the learners believe that positive actions will make them successful, and the learners select outcomes to believe NLP made things possible (Hutton; 2017).

To summarise Dr, Bandler expressed in the public domain that the brand name NLP sounded smart; hence there is no secret agenda. NLP research is underdeveloped, a small number of an academic article is available, and most of the pieces of evidence are non-empirical. NLP governance is weak, and there is no universal regulation in order. NLP certifications have inconsistent criteria, varying study modules, titles, and requirements (Dr. Kotera, Y).

In conclusion, despite NLP's success, it is not seen as a scientific method. Perhaps an international regulatory body of NLP society, creating strict criteria of NLP study modules underlying a set of universal requirements for the practitioners and equipping of field and academic research on the strategies and effect of NLP on the subjects (clients) will help to generate further academic papers to examine its validity and scientific approaches.

References

Benefits and Work Guides You Can Trus; https://www.benefitsandwork.co.uk/; From https://www.benefitsandwork.co.uk/news/3113-; 10 June 2015; Accessed on 20 July 2021

Dr. Kotera, Yasuhiro; University of Derby; NLP: Why this therapy has failed to join the mainstream; https://www.derby.ac.uk/; from https://www.derby.ac.uk/blog/neuro-linguistic-programming-psychology/; Accessed on 23 July 2021

Good Therapy; https://www.goodtherapy.org/; Neuro-Linguistic Programming (NLP); from https://www.goodtherapy.org/learn-about-therapy/types/neuro-linguistic-programming; Accessed on 20 July 2021

Hutton, G; Myths of NLP; https://mindpersuasion.com/; from https://mindpersuasion.com/myths-of-nlp/#comments; 21 October 2017; Accessed on 20 July 2021

The Society of Medical NLP™; from https://www.medicalnlp.com/about-us/; Accessed on 19 July 2021

Thomson, Garner; Khan, Khalid; Magic in Practice Introducing Medical NLP: The Art and Science of Language in Healing and Health; Hammersmith Press LTD; 2008)

Williams, Cassi; Transformational NLP; The spiritual approach to harnessing the power of Neuro-Linguistic Programming; Watkins Publishing; 2012

PSYCHOLOGY

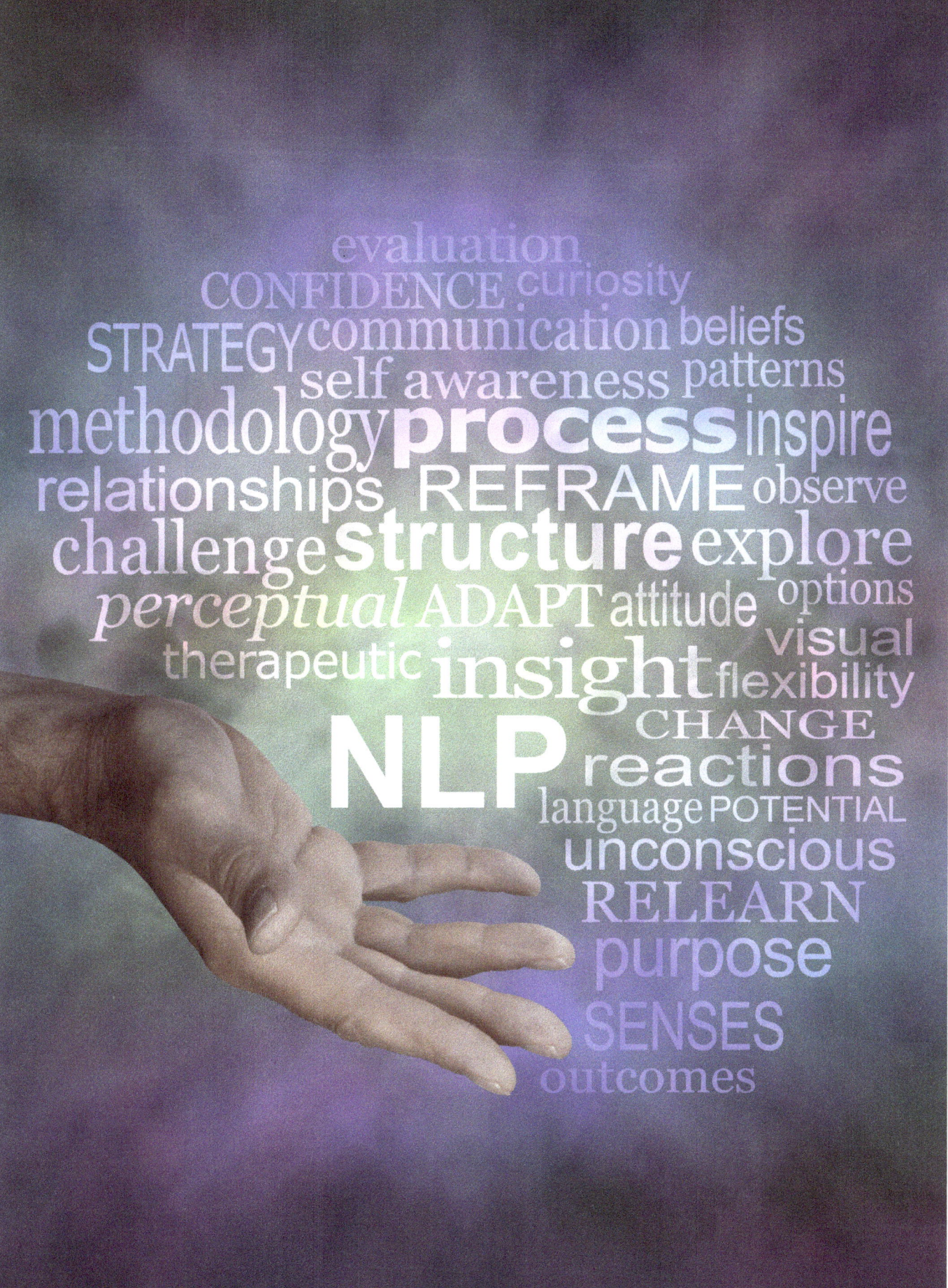

PHARMACOLOGY

HOW DO ANTIDEPRESSANTS WORK?

> Pharmacology   > by: Dr Ahmad Saeed

Depression, anxiety, SAD, and dysthymia (a minor form of persistent depression) may all be treated with antidepressants. Taking an antidepressant may be a component of your therapy for depression. Antidepressants' precise mechanism of action is a mystery.

Various substances are used by our brain's nerve cells to transmit messages. Even though many aspects are still unknown, scientists think that depression is caused by an imbalance of certain chemical messengers (neurotransmitters), such as serotonin, which means that messages cannot be effectively transmitted through the nerves as intended. Antidepressants are designed to make these substances more readily available. Different medicines work in different ways to do this.

Antidepressants may alleviate depression's symptoms, but they don't always go to the root of the problem. Therefore antidepressants are often used in conjunction with therapy to combat more severe forms of depression or other mental health issues. When you take an antidepressant, your brain's chemical messengers, known as neurotransmitters, are restored to their normal balance. These antidepressants may help lift your spirits, enhance your sleep, and boost your energy and focus.

A professional psychologist in Boston believes antidepressants may assist in jump-starting a person's mood and give them the push they need to overcome their depression symptoms. A more optimistic outlook is a result of "this frequently allowing them to start doing the things they love again and make better choices for themselves." Taking an antidepressant is a big decision, and it's essential to be prepared.

Effectiveness

Antidepressants may be beneficial for individuals who are suffering from mild to severe depression, according to the available research. For individuals with certain illnesses, studies have demonstrated that they're better than a placebo ("dummy medication"). Unless other therapies like counselling have failed, they are seldom suggested for moderate depression.

Forms of Antidepressants

Tablets are the most common delivery method for antidepressants. If you're given these drugs, you'll begin treatment with the smallest dosage deemed necessary to alleviate your condition.

Before feeling the effects of an antidepressant, you generally must take it for one to two weeks (without skipping a dosage). Take them as prescribed, and don't stop taking them if you have any minor side effects at first.

Consult your primary care provider or a mental health professional if you've been on an antidepressant for four weeks and haven't noticed any improvement. It's possible that they'll suggest upping your dosage or switching to a different medication.

A therapy program is typically completed in a span of six months or more. Recurrent depression may necessitate the recommendation that some individuals take antidepressants for an extended period.

When are Antidepressants needed?

Antidepressants may or may not be a choice, depending on a variety of factors, such as the severity of the patient's symptoms. Other factors may come into play while making a choice:

Are you currently in treatment, or do you have any plans to attend?

What previous antidepressants have you tried, and how have they worked for you?

Do you believe the probable negative consequences outweigh the positive ones?

When selecting a medication, consideration should be given to possible adverse effects. Some individuals may be more concerned with keeping their digestive system in good working order than others. Some men may want to avoid experiencing side effects, including dizziness, reduced sexual desire, or troublesome erections altogether.

Antidepressants should only be used if the underlying diagnosis is accurate. Antidepressants are given to certain patients even though they don't need them, according to medical experts. The fact that antidepressants are being used by so many more individuals nowadays indicates that this is correct. Even though it's not known whether they assist with minor depression, they're occasionally already given for modest symptoms.

However, it's critical to appropriately identify and treat severe depression if it's present. Anxiolytics may assist here and, for some individuals, maybe the only option is to return to everyday life or start going to psychotherapy.

Other considerations may come into play if you're expecting a child. Antidepressants should be used with caution by pregnant women.

Important things to keep in mind

Taking antidepressant medication together with therapy may help you get your life back on track. A change in lifestyle and counseling may be all you require if your symptoms are minor.

Taking antidepressants is nothing to be embarrassed about. Depression is a medical condition, not a fault or weakness of character. Your personality will not be altered by the medications.

It takes time for antidepressants to take effect. To be honest, you may have to test several different things before you discover one that works well.

People quit using antidepressants for a variety of reasons. However, seek medical advice. There are many methods for dealing with adverse effects. Also, reducing the dosage or switching medications may be beneficial.

Long-term medication use is a frightening prospect. However, many individuals may gradually wean themselves off antidepressants over time.

Antidepressants vs. Hypnotherapy

In addition to antidepressant medication and cognitive-behavioral therapy, hypnotherapy has been studied as a treatment for depression. Patients' pulse rate, respiration, and blood pressure fall during hypnotherapy sessions because they are moved into deeper states of awareness. It's possible for patients who've attained the deepest degree of consciousness to remember and feel things they'd previously blocked from their awareness.

"The hypnotherapist helps the patient build new, healthier thinking processes and habits to utilize when mentally facing depressed situations," explains the statement.

Depression is a problem that a lot of people are having to cope with these days. Anxiety, tension, and sorrow are all terms that individuals use to describe this feeling. In a general opinion, and in terms of hypnotherapy, the name doesn't matter all that much.

What's alarming is the rise in the number of individuals taking antidepressants or being urged to do so by their doctors.

In many instances, this medicine is necessary and helpful for the patient, and physicians can be trusted to recognize these scenarios. When this occurs, it's important to be on board with their usage and to defer to the expertise of our medical experts.

As a result, there are a few things to be worried about.

When it comes to widely given antidepressants, "researchers, who have released a study analyzing the effect of the medicines on the whole body, believe they seem to be doing patients more damage than good."

Second, even though antidepressants are widely used and have serious side effects, only 30 to 50 percent of individuals seem to benefit from them.

People who are depressed frequently seek assistance from their doctor but leave with little more than a prescription in hand.

Again, hypnotherapy may be the best option for many of these patients. Antidepressants may be the sole option for someone whose brain chemistry is permanently and substantially out of balance.

Pharmacogenomics of Antidepressant Drugs

Depression is a significant public health issue, affecting 5–10 percent of women and 2–5 percent of men. For women, the lifetime risk is 10–25 percent, while for men, it is 5–12 percent. When it comes to treating the major depressive disorder and anxiety disorders, antidepressants are extensively utilized. However, only half of the patients react to antidepressant therapy, and only a third of patients see improvement. A variety of pharmacogenomic variables influence the way antidepressants and other CNS medications work, including their pharmacodynamics as well as their pharmacokinetics. CYP enzymes are involved in the metabolism of most antidepressants.

Atypical antidepressants are among the most often given medications in the industrialized world. There is over 60% variability in antidepressant pharmacodynamic and pharmacokinetics due to pharmacogenomics (including selective serotonin reuptake inhibitors, serotonin-norepinephrine reuptake inhibitors, tricyclic and tetra-cycle compounds, monoamine oxidase inhibitors, and noradrenaline- and serotonin-modulators). Five major categories of genes are involved in the pharmacogenomic response to antidepressant drugs. These are:

Genes linked to depression pathogenesis

Genes linked to drug mechanism of action

Genes linked to drug metabolism

Genes linked to drug transporters

Pleiotropic genes involved in multiple cascades and metabolic reactivity

The main substrates of the CYP1A2 enzymes include around 24% of antidepressants, 5% of CYP2B6, 38% of CYP2C19, 85% of CYP2D6, and 38% of CYP3A4. About a quarter of Caucasians are weak in the CYP2D6-CYP2C19-CYP2C9 cluster's enzyme activity, which is responsible for the metabolism of 60% of currently available medications. The application of pharmacogenomic techniques in the therapeutic environment may assist mental patients in getting the most benefit from their antidepressant medication.

Prescription of antidepressants through trial and error, ignoring the pharmacogenetic profile of patients, is susceptible to a 60 percent mistake rate with concomitant issues in effectiveness and safety, according to recent research, according to recent studies reveal.

Pharmacogenetics' therapeutic teachings in the past included the following:

The effects of drugs differ from person to person and are affected by genetics in some way.

Most medication reactions have several causes.

Drug-metabolizing enzymes are affected by numerous genetic polymorphisms of single genes

It is becoming clearer that genetic variations in drug targets and drug transporters are to blame for the wide range of pharmacological reactions.

Treatment is only effective in subgroups of individuals who have sensitizing mutations in one or more of the targeted proteins

There are substantial ethnic differences in medication effects, whether multifactorial or hereditary

The use of response-predictive genetic profiles on clinical outcomes has been limited to research institutions and has not yet made it into clinical use.

References

Depression: Should I Take an Antidepressant? | HealthLink BC. (2019, May 28). HealthLink BC. https://www.healthlinkbc.ca/health-topics/ty6745.

Depression: How Effective Are Antidepressants? – InformedHealth.org – NCBI Bookshelf. (2020, June 18). https://www.ncbi.nlm.nih.gov/books/NBK361016/.

Overview – Antidepressants – NHS. (n.d.). nhs.uk.

https://www.nhs.uk/mental-health/talking-therapies-medicine-treatments/medicines-and-psychiatry/antidepressants/overview/.

Antidepressants: Types, Side Effects, Uses, And Effectiveness. (n.d.). https://www.medicalnewstoday.com/articles/248320#_noHeaderPrefixedContent.

How Antidepressants and Depression Medication Can Affect Your Life. (2010, July 9). WebMD. https://www.webmd.com/depression/features/antidepressant-effects.

Depression And Hypnotherapy – Nichols Clinical Hypnotherapy. (n.d.). http://nicholsclinicalhypnotherapy.com/depression-antidepressants-hypnotherapy.

TRANSCRANIAL DIRECT CURRENT STIMULATION

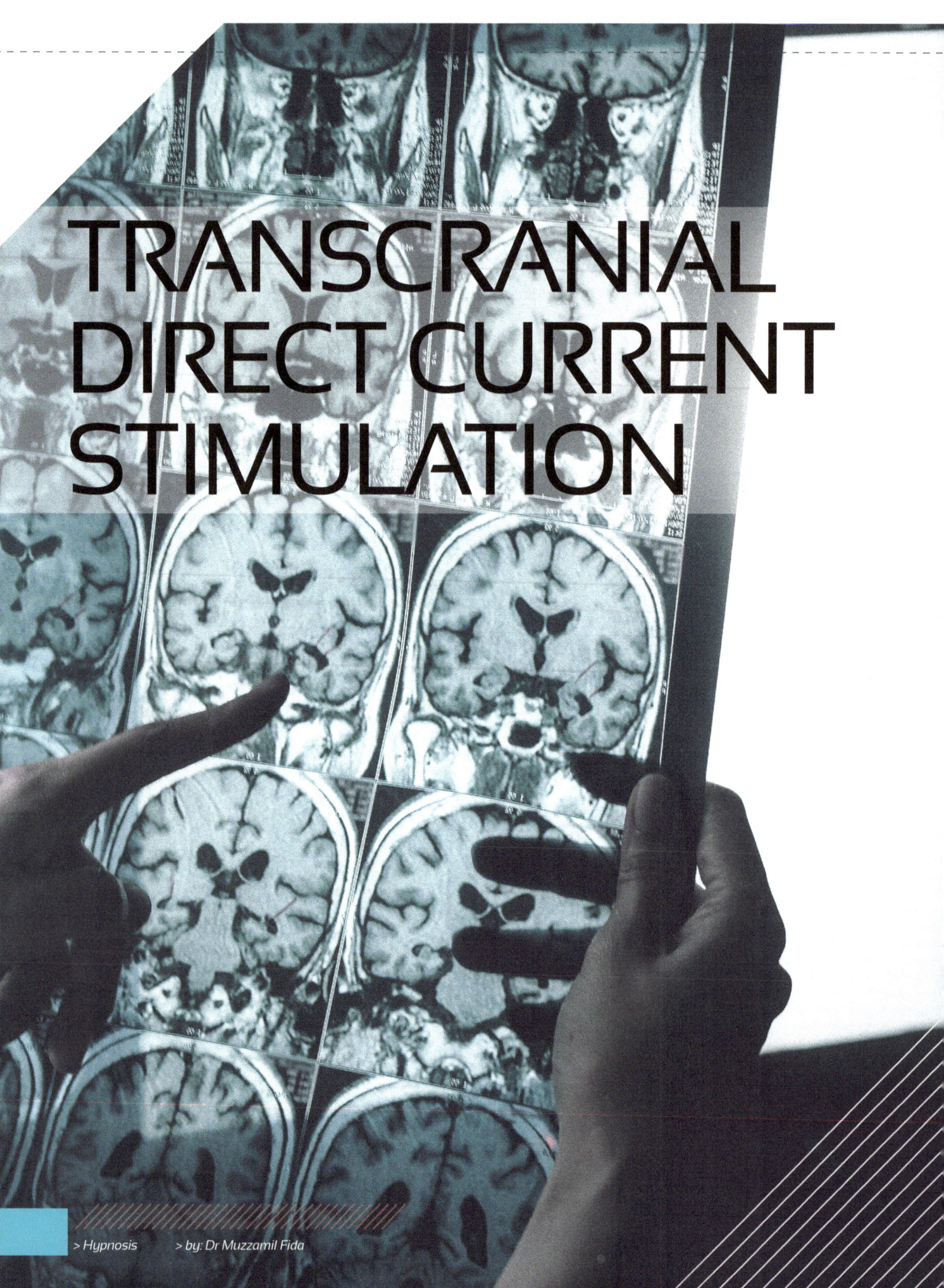

> Hypnosis   > by: Dr Muzzamil Fida

Transcranial
direct current stimulation

It is the use of direct electrical currents to stimulate specific areas in the brain. The process is painless and does not need any surgery. The electrodes are placed on the head, and the low-frequency current is passed to change the neuronal activity (Elsner et al., 2017).

Here are the pros and cons of the transcranial direct current stimulation (tDCS):

Pros:

It improves the learning process of the brain. The cognitive function is also enhanced. The primary motor cortex significantly enhances the motor skill task if it is stimulated by tDCS.

The driving abilities improve after stimulating the dorsolateral prefrontal cortex.

The cortical regions such as the primary and secondary somatosensory cortex and anterior cingulate cortex are linked with pain perception. Therefore, tDCS is also used to treat some chronic pain conditions which are unresponsive to any other medication or medication used to have serious side effects such as fibromyalgia – in this condition, opioids are used, which cause severe side effects (K, 2012).

The language learning skills are improved when the left frontal lobe of the brain is stimulated.

The two-week therapy is helpful in patients suffering from depression. The stimulation in the left dorsolateral prefrontal cortex increases the cortical function and helps in depression.

It is used to improve sleep quality by increasing the time of the deep and profound phases of sleep. For this reason, it is used in post-polio syndrome to improve quality of the sleep.

In attention-deficit/hyperactivity disorder, tDCS is helpful to focus selectively and increase attention.

The stimulation of the motor cortex of the brain can be helpful in patients with stroke (Elsner et al., 2017). The stroke-induced aphasia is corrected by tDCS.

The working memory and cognitive functions are significantly improved by stimulating the dorsolateral prefrontal cortex (DLPFC) region by tDCS. The excitability of this region increases the performance.

It also enhances visual attention.

Cons

Mild tingling, burning, and itching sensation is felt at the point of the electrode. The transcranial direct current stimulation-induced erythema can alter the binding and intensity of the electrodes.

Headache and nausea occur due to stimulation of the chemoreceptor trigger zone in the brain by the current.

Some patients have insomnia due to changes in cortical stimulation.

Regular use of the electrodes causes transcranial direct current stimulation-induced erythema, which can be severe. The erythema is reduced by pre-treating the skin with ketoprofen, hydroxyzine, and lidocaine.

The direct current is affected by the media present in ways such as hair that can play the role of an insulator. Therefore, the use of saline water is needed.

The current is also affected by sweat. The sweat is a conductor due to which the current intensity changes.

The transcranial direct current stimulation is also reported to change some complex behavior such as impulsivity.

Transcranial direct current stimulation and hypnosis in treating depression

Several studies show that in the treatment of depression, transcranial direct current stimulation is very effective in treating depression (Moffa et al., 2020). In transcranial direct current stimulation, a direct current of 1-2 mA is applied, which may cause alteration in the cortical excitability. The effects last for a few hours, and the continuous stimulation causes changes in the synaptic connections. The therapeutic effect of the stimulation in depression is achieved through the release of neurotransmitters. However, the exact efficacy of the tDCS is still not understood, and further investigation is required. Another prevalent method to treat depression is the use of hypnosis (Rosa & Lisanby, 2012). While patients are remaining in the hypnotic state, they target the unnecessary and unhealthy habits and learn to control them (Hypnotherapy and Depression: How It Works, n.d.). During hypnosis, the connection between the dorsolateral prefrontal cortex and insula increases. This does not involve any medications and devices, while in tDCS, electrodes are used to stimulate the mentioned area.

References

Elsner, B., Kwakkel, G., Kugler, J., & Mehrholz, J. (2017). Transcranial direct current stimulation (tDCS) for improving capacity in activities and arm function after stroke: a network meta-analysis of randomised controlled trials. Journal of NeuroEngineering and Rehabilitation, 14(1), 95. https://doi.org/10.1186/s12984-017-0301-7

Hypnotherapy and Depression: How it Works. (n.d.). Retrieved October 30, 2021, from https://www.healthline.com/health/depression/hypnotherapy

K, L. (2012). Transcranial direct current stimulation for the reduction of clinical and experimentally induced pain: a systematic review and meta-analysis. Clin J Pain, 28(5), 452–461. https://doi.org/10.1097/AJP.0b013e31823853e3

Moffa, A. H., Martin, D., Alonzo, A., Bennabi, D., Blumberger, D. M., Benseñor, I. M., Daskalakis, Z., Fregni, F., Haffen, E., Lisanby, S. H., & Padberg, F. (2020). Efficacy and acceptability of transcranial direct current stimulation (tDCS) for major depressive disorder: An individual patient data meta-analysis. Progress in Neuro-Psychopharmacology and Biological Psychiatry, 99, 109836. https://doi.org/10.1016/j.pnpbp.2019.109836

Rosa, M., & Lisanby, S. (2012). Somatic treatments for mood disorders. Neuropsychopharmacology, 37(1), 102–116. https://doi.org/10.1038/npp.2011.225

HYPNOTHERAPY

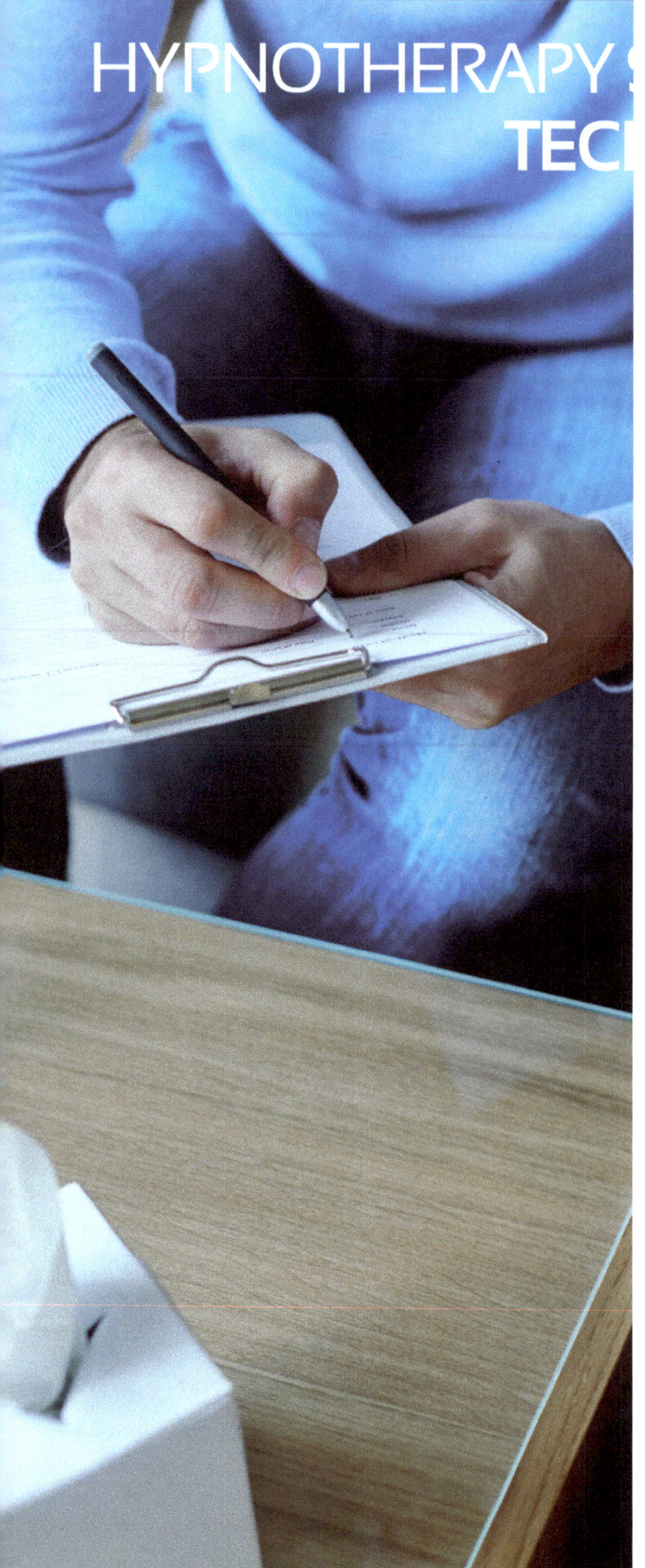

HYPNOTHERAPY SPECIALIZATIONS, TECHNIQUES & TOOLS

> Hypnotherapy   > by: Shanta Sultana   > e: shanta.sultana@hypnosis.plus

Hypnosis is an altered and yet natural state of the conscious mind that can be naturally used for therapeutic purposes with the option to amend unwanted habits and behaviours. Hypnosis is a type of psychotherapy. It is generally described as an altered state of the conscious mind. However, hypnosis is a phenomenon that is still being studied.

The purpose of this article is to list a certain number of hypnotherapy tools, techniques and specializations. We shall begin with what is Clinical hypnotherapy and why it is important.

HYPNOTHERAPY

Clinical Hypnotherapy (specialization): Clinical hypnotherapy means using advanced methods of hypnosis and other techniques to treat a variety of medical and psychological problems and upwards of 85 per cent of people will readily respond to clinical hypnotherapy.

Clinical hypnotherapy is an advanced field in hypnotherapy that treats various medical and psychological problems, acknowledged as a complementary treatment and recognized by the British Medical Association (BMA) in 1955. In 1958, The American Psychological Association (APA) approved it. Today the NHS and many official medical societies globally recognize it (British Society of Clinical Hypnosis).

The effects of hypnotherapy are different based on each subject, and hypnotherapists use a variety of techniques and tools depending on what works best to treat the symptoms. So, let's have a comprehensive look at some hypnotherapy techniques, tools and specializations.

Suggestion Hypnotherapy (it is considered to be traditional hypnotherapy - specialization): During hypnosis, a brain scan has shown the shifts of brainwave from Beta State[1] to Alpha State[2]. This is similar to the way the brain behaves in the state of relaxation or meditation. In this state, our subconscious mind is perceptive to take suggestions. The hypnotist will put suggestions based on the reason the client has sought help (Hypnotherapy Directory).

Direct Suggestion (technique): is perhaps the most common technique, in which the hypnotherapist suggests the desired behaviour. It requires minimal mental activity from the client's perspective, so it may suit particular personalities. It is effective when the session is repeated multiple times (Moving Minds).

Indirect Suggestion (technique): gives control to the client, and it is often a favourite method for hypnotherapists. It is more effective for those who are sceptical of trance. The therapist does not order the client but might request, "You might wish to close your eyes when you are comfortable." This was the favourite method for Milton Erickson. (Brooks, S.; British Hypnosis Research).

Ericksonian Hypnotherapy (specialization): Milton Erickson (1901-1980; Nevada, USA) discovered indirect suggestions. Direct suggestion suggests the subjects enter hypnosis or how to alter the undesirable patterns of behaviour. Indirect suggestion looks like: "You might wish to discuss the alternatives to eating if you are ready to do so." He created an approach that was different and new and can be classified as an existential approach. Erickson did not see the client's history as the focal point; he used metaphors, anecdotes, contradictions, and symbols, resulting in important behavioural changes. His questions were with detailed inquiry and would express genuine interest in the client. Ericksonian techniques and strategies include Interpersonal, Nonverbal (also known as Pantomime tactics), and Handshake Hypnotic Induction technique so-called the Ericksonian approach comes under the Utilization Approach.

Cognitive Hypnotherapy (specialization): Helps to update the subconsciousness in line with the consciousness and the client's understanding of reality. Here, hypnosis is assimilated with Cognitive Behavioural Therapy. In cognitive therapy, behaviours are based on early experiences; hence explicit negative experiences influence the negative thoughts, emotions, and behaviour. Behaviour Therapy says that negative behaviour is self-taught; therefore, it can be unlearned. Incorporating hypnosis increases the motivation level establishing positive cognitions that may act on the conscious state and positive imaging and suggestion that may make those positive behavioural changes (Hypnotherapy Directory & D'Souza, R.; Clinical Hypnotherapy Cardiff).

Hypnoanalysis (technique): The concepts are drawn from psychotherapy, and the roots of the triggers and the causes of the current problems are identified. The practitioner works after identifying the root causes; hence this technique involves more sessions than other methods. It uses the psychoanalytic theory that past events often cause the current problems. The client shares things from the past. However, the client may provide all details under hypnosis. The subconscious mind stores information, hence, hypnosis allows the subconscious to reveal them. Once desirable information is found, new ways of thinking or behaviour may be suggested. (Hypnotherapy Directory and D'Souza, R.; Clinical Hypnotherapy Cardiff).

Age Regression (technique): The subject gradually travels back in time how it is necessary. People describe their experience under this technique as an interesting experience. The subject may call sad or traumatic experiences and react. (Farthing; 1992).

Criticism: The theory is controversial because there is not enough research available to support it and claim that it may embed false memories. (The Good Therapy) It has also been debated that not all Regression therapy is helpful, especially when the therapist is biased about the client's history (D'Souza, R.; Clinical Hypnotherapy Cardiff).

Dr. Julia Shaw's research suggests that complex memories can be generated under regression techniques. Participants may remember things that never happened. These are called "Rich False Memories" and the subject's life in the real world can be badly affected by these memories. Dr. Shaw says that these memories are easy to generate as most people accept the idea of repression. (Shaw, J; Scientific American).

Under hypnosis, the subject may report some accurate events but may also report many false memories. Hypnosis may increase the confidence of the subject to report events without increasing the accuracy level of the memory. Leading questions, with or without under the hypnotic influence can lead the subject to agree. (Ferthing, 1992; Berkeley; Shaw, J; Scientific American)

Cognitive-Behavioural Hypnotherapy (specialization): Cognitive Behavioural Hypnotherapy uses Cognitive therapeutic techniques along with a number of theories such as Positive Psychology, Neuroscience and NLP. It incorporates hypnosis to help the subconscious to update in line with the conscious. It gives the client control over feelings, thoughts and behaviours. It is the subconscious that tries to keep the subject safe by seeing and feeling in a certain way. Cognitive Hypnotherapy helps to change the way the subject behaves or feels towards a problematic area. (Hypnotherapy Directory).

Solution Focused Hypnotherapy (specialization): Looks for positive change instead of focusing on the problem. The philosophy is based on the works of Steve De Shazer and Insoo Kim Berg. They developed Solution Focused Brief Therapy or SFBT, and it is used in psychotherapy and hypnotherapy. In this method, the client is set with a goal; at a deep state of relaxation, the client is more susceptible to suggestions and guided imaginations, making achieving the goal possible. Hence this is the difference between SFBT and Solution Focused Hypnotherapy (Hypnotherapy Directory).

Solution Focused Hypnotherapy is concerned with the resolution instead of the problem. It uses a scaling in which the subject identifies where they are. This helps to move forward and map a progress plan. It believes that each client is unique therefore, the service is specifically mapped for the client's needs. The goals set are to achieve a solution and the clients can self-assess the result on themselves. (Hypnotherapy Directory)

Guided Imagery (tool): This is effective because of the mind and body connection. The therapist prompts the subject to focus on a scene on which the subject notices various sensory aspects. The guided imagery tool involves all five senses hence the subject can smell, hear or feel the texture of something. Hence, it affects the body and mind.

I.e. With pain relief treatment, the subject is asked to imagine something pleasant. Thus, a tailored storyline with visual images can be created for the subject to re-enter the pleasant place. The most

HYPNOTHERAPY

effective images are with those that have senses, such as smell, touch, or taste. It can help with pain management, post-operative conditions, and asthma. This method is particularly effective for children to have a vivid imagination and be taught self-hypnosis in under an hour. It can also be effective online or over the telephone. Hypnosis is incorporating the Guided Imagery tool, can utilize the relaxed state to help a person become more receptive to new ideas and beliefs; it can utilise the subject's senses to better direct and focus attention on a particular area of concern, i.e. the subject can imagine the desired outcome (Good Therapy).

Stop Technique: Thoughts occur about future events; however, some of those thoughts are erroneous, and they can impair the subject's mood and practical abilities to self-improvement. The right kind of worry is necessary to accomplish something; therefore, first, the unnecessary thoughts are to be filtered out (exposure) and ask if these thoughts should be stopped. The therapist gives certain breathing techniques, physical tasks, such as specific physical exercise, i.e., jaw exercise when the subject is worried about public speaking, and mental images to stop the negative thoughts, such as squeezing the thought into a fist (Wallace, C; Blooming Lotus Hypnosis).

Parts Therapy (technique): The human mind is split into many different elements. Each of them has its own function. To look at the simple daily tasks such as walk, talk, eat, drive and countless other daily tasks, it is apparent that our brain does all these things simultaneously. Sometimes a part of the human mind does not work at the same pace. I.e. when someone says "A part of me can't follow this diet". This can hold someone back from making a positive change. The mind is functioning by establishing learned behaviours to protect whereas, in fact, it has an adverse effect on the subject. For example, procrastination: the subject wants to start the task to make a positive change. But the brain thinks it is protecting the subject by holding him back. Parts Hypnotherapy empowers the client to explore different parts of the brain and find solutions. The client is in a hypnotic state and the subconscious responds to the hypnotherapist's suggestions often with signals such as with a movement of a finger or hand. The client is fully aware of what is happening. (Hypnotherapy Directory).

Mindfulness in Hypnotherapy (tool): Effective when combined with hypnotherapy. Mindfulness is a state of active, open attention to the present. It helps to manage stress and anxiety. It is a non-judgemental awareness.

TimeLine Therapy (TTL) (technique): The positive effect of TTL is known to be more retainable than other forms of therapy. TTL learns from past events and uses these as resources to help the client remove negative emotions, such as anger, sadness, guilt, and fear. TTL was developed by the NLP practitioner Dr. Tad James. It has been successfully used since 1986 by psychologists, social workers, counsellors, and life coaches (TimeLine Therapy®). TTL is not hypnotherapy itself, but it is combined with hypnosis. It is also called brief therapy. TTL believes that we unconsciously store a mental photo album following a timeline. TTL helps the client overcome the limitation that was set by the past negative emotions and project on the positive future (Hypnotherapy Directory and D'Souza, R.; Clinical Hypnotherapy Cardiff; TimeLine Therapy®).

Rapid Transformational Therapy (RTT) (specialization): Combines NLP, hypnotherapy, and psychotherapy. It was created by celebrity therapist and hypnotherapist trainer Marisa Peer. It puts the client in deep relaxation and a perceptive state and uses a form of regression therapy to have hypnotic conditioning (alter thought process and behaviour). As a result, the clients are in a heightened state of focus & control and get trained to connect with the subconscious. (Hypnotherapy Directory).

Hypno-Psychotherapy (specialization): When multiple branches of psychotherapy such as but not limited to psychodynamic Humanist, Gestalt, and mindfulness are integrated. The practitioners are trained in these branches to apply Hypno-Psychotherapy; hence they differ from hypnotherapists. The benefit is the client can make sense of controlling emotions and what triggers them. This specialization is good for complex emotional, psychological, and practitioners may state that only psychotherapy would not have the same result. It also helps to have other medical applications such as post-operative treatments, pain relief strategies, and anaesthesia and assist with migraine, skin disorders, and IBS (D'Souza, R.; Clinical Hypnotherapy Cardiff).

Gestalt therapy (specialization): Gestalt was developed by Fritz Perls and his wife in the 1940s. It gives attention to how to make a sense of the world and experiences. It is a form of psychotherapy that is focusing on the present instead of exploring the past. It focuses on taking responsibility. This also involves role play where the client speaks with another part of the mind or with another person in real or not. Body language is observed by the therapist and sometimes creative art is used.

Combining the Gestalt approach with hypnotherapy is a highly effective way to help the client reach the desired place. It helps the client see things immediately instead of over-intellectualizing and generating too much emotion (Farahani, R. G.; Gestalt Ottowa; Kraft, D; London Psychotherapy).

Neuro-Linguistic Programming (NLP) (tool): NLP gives the perspective to the client to overcome obstacles. NLP was created by two American academics, Dr. Richard Bandler and John Grinder, in the 70s, who saw the relationship between language behaviour and excellence. They saw:

Neuro- All of our experiences are gained from the neurological process that rules our five senses; taste, touch, smell, sight, and sound.

Linguistic- We interpret our experiences through a set of filters, including languages. The language we use affects our experiences.

Programming- The way to control or create a path to excellence. By adjusting the language, the person can be in the "pre-excellence" category.

People's limitations in thought processes are deeply embedded in the subconscious mind. Using NLP, the hypnotherapist can alter the thought pattern. The hypnotherapist looks at the language used, the language patterns, the attitude, and emotional & physical state; he or she will also assess and analyse to create a strategy to improve motivation, learning abilities, and how positive memories and imaginations can be formed (Hypnotherapy Directory).

Kappasian Hypnosis Model (specialization): Dr. John G. Kappas (1925-2002), the American hypnotist, redefined hypnosis and created his revolutionary model - "Message Unit Theory" and "Emotional and Physical Suggestibility and Sexuality" Theory, which help to understand human behaviour and responses in a deeper and comprehensive level and assist in finding solutions for the subject. Many see him as the father of hypnosis, and he made it possible to distinguish hypnotherapy as a profession separated from Psychotherapy. He authored the definition of Hypnotist and Hypnotherapist in the Federal Dictionary of Occupational Titles, and in 1973, the profession had official recognition. Dr. Kappas practised for thirty-two years until his death, taught and wrote books, and created a manual for hypnotism. Dr. Kappas's biggest contribution to hypnosis is the "E&P" model. They are Emotional and Physical Suggestibility and Emotional and Physical sexuality. They belong to the Kappasian School of Hypnotism. Based on this, suggestibility assessments are created. Physically suggestible minds tend to process input literally, and Emotionally suggestible minds are analytical and prefer an indirect approach. Nevertheless, no one falls in one category hundred per cent though it is dominated by one category than the other. Using these models, the hypnotherapist can also analyse the language pattern the subject uses (Perin, R; Hypnothechs).

Dynamic Hypnosis (tool): Dynamic hypnosis uses "sign and gesture".

HYPNOTHERAPY

Therefore, non-verbal and symbolic communication acts at a deep level that controls the emotional sphere of the individual hence the client get to know self. It enables the client to listen to their own body and mind. The client is able to find the background of the problem and anticipate solutions (Brown & Fromm; 2009).

This was a basic guide to various specializations, tools and techniques in hypnotherapy. Readers are encouraged to research and explore further and involve in studies if interested in the practice or receive treatment with any of the mentioned techniques.

Perhaps you would like to add some comments, techniques, specializations that you think should not have been missed in this list, please send it via email at info@ihypnosis.plus

[1] Beta Wave: Associated with the normal waking conscious state

[2] Alpha Wave: A state of wakeful relaxation. A person is calmer and less anxious in this state. Some studies say this state boost creativity levels.

References

Andrade G. (2017). Is past life regression therapy ethical? Journal of medical ethics and history of medicine, 10, 11. ; Retrieved from https://www.ncbi.nlm.nih.gov/pmc/articles/PMC5797677/; Retrieved on 14 June 2021

Barabasz, A and Watkins, J. G; 2005; Hypnotheraputic Techniques; Brunner-Routledge

Brooks, Stephen; 2021; English; British Hypnosis Research & Training Institute; British Hypnosis Research; Retrieved on 14 June 2021; From https://britishhypnosisresearch.com/hypnosis-techniques/

Brown, D.P; Fromm, E; 2009; Hypnotherapy and Hypnoalalysis; First edition 1948; Routledge

British Society of Clinical Hypnosis (ND); Retrieved June 14, 2021; From https://www.bsch.org.uk

D'Souza, Richard; 2021; F.P.R.M.S; J A Cardiff; Clinical Hypnotherapy Cardiff; Retrieved on 14 June 2021; https://www.clinicalhypnotherapy-cardiff.co.uk/types-of-hypnotherapy/

Farhani, Razi, Ghaemmagham; Welcome at Gestalt Ottwa (ND); Gestalt and Hypnosis; retrieved June 14, 2021; https://gestaltottawa.com/; https://gestaltottawa.com/wp-content/uploads/2012/08/Gestalt-Hypnosis.pdf; Retrieved on June 14 2021

Ferthing, W, G; The Psychology of Consciousness; 1992; https://www.ocf.berkeley.edu/; Hypnotic Age Regression and Hypermnesia; From https://www.ocf.berkeley.edu/~jfkihlstrom/ConsciousnessWeb/Farthing/Chapter16.pdf; Retrieved on 02 July 2021

Good Therapy; Find The Right Therapist (ND); Regression Therapy; Retrieved June 14, 2021; From https://www.goodtherapy.org/

Good Therapy; Guided Therapeutic Imagery (ND); https://goodtherapy.org/; From https://www.goodtherapy.org/learn-about-therapy/types/guided-therapeutic-imagery; Retrieved on June 14, 2021

Good Therapy; Cognitive Behavioural Therapy (CBT); https://goodtherapy.org/; From: https://www.goodtherapy.org/learn-about-therapy/types/cognitive-behavioral-therapy; Retrieved on July 10 2021

Hypnosis (ND); Hypnozine; Hypnosis Magazine; Retrieved June 14 2021; From https://hypnozine.com/humanist-hypnosis/

Hypnotherapy Directory; Find Hypnotherapist Near You; English; J. Chapman; J. Hollingsworth; A. Jackson; Retrieved on 14 June 2021; From https://www.hypnotherapy-directory.org.uk/content/hypnotherapy-types.html

Jong; Boers; Wietmarchen; Tromp; Bousari; Wannekes; Snoeck; Bekhof; Vlieger; Springer (ND); Hypnotherapy or transcendental meditation versus progressive muscle relaxation exercises in the treatment of children with primary headaches: a multi-centre, pragmatic, randomised clinical study; 2018; Retrieved 14 June 2021; From https://link.springer.com

Kraft, D; London Psychotherapy; www.londonpsychotherapy.co.uk; Journal of Integrative Research, Counselling and Psychotherapy, vol.2, no.1; The Relevance of Gestalt Therapy To Clinicians Who Use Hypnosis Today; February 2016; From https://www.londonhypnotherapyuk.com/publications/Gestalt-Therapy-Paper.pdf; Retrieved on 14 June 2021

Past Life Regression (ND); The Past Life Therapist Association; Retrieved; June 14 2021; From https://www.pastliferegression.co.k/index.html

Perin, R; Hypnotechs, Clinical Hypnotherapy; Kappasian Hypnosis; https://resources.hypnotechs.com/theory-mind; Retrieved on 14 June 2021

TimeLine Therapy®.; NLP Coaching & TimeLine Therapy; English; Tad James Company; Retrieved on 14 June 2021; From https://www.nlpcoaching.com/time-line-therapy/

Wallace, C; Blooming Lotus Hypnosis; Stop Intrusive Thoughts; https://www.bloominglotushypnosis.com/wellness-campaign/2020/2/20/stop-intrusive-thoughts

Zimberoff, D and Hartman, D; The Wellness Institute (ND); The Heart-Centred Hypnotherapy Modality Defined; Retrieved June 14, 2021; From https://www.wellness-institute.org/

Zimberoff, D; The Wellness Institute (ND); Five Principals of Existential Hypnotherapy 2013; Retrieved on June 14; From https://web.wellness-institute.org/blog/bid/353582/five-principles-of-existential-hypnotherapy

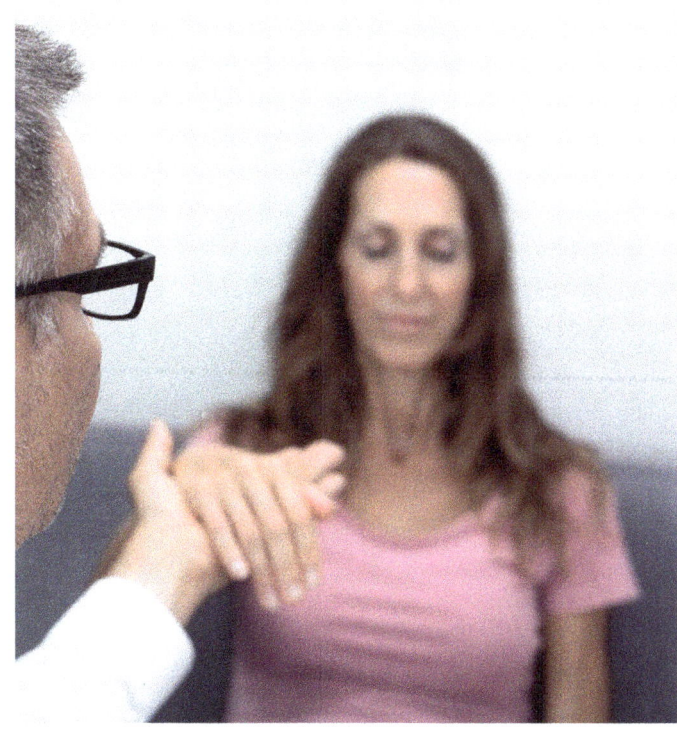

PSYCHOLOGY

HOW
AND
AS AN

> Special feature
> by: Shanta Sultana

PSYCHOLOGY

TO DEFEAT THE PANDEMIC
COME OUT ACHIEVER

With guides from Mike Pegg

"There is nothing, no clues. I don't know what is going to happen; what can you actually do, what are you doing?" A friend of mine asked me in March 2020 when she was laid off from an international company where she had been serving as a senior worker for years. I asked her if she could think of something else she could actually do and maybe work with that. Her immediate answer was she did not have any skills. After a conversation, I understood, by other skills, she was thinking of a major qualification such as IT or Accounting. When I explained that it could be something she practiced as a hobby, she found my thoughts childish at first. Interestingly, she started practicing yoga in the park last summer, something she was able to offer to other women during the isolation. Until now, she never thought of herself as a mind and body health instructor. She was raised to think she needed to be in an office to be a validated working woman. This is what the pandemic has done. It has changed the whole dynamic of how we need to think and see the world.

This isn't necessarily a bad thing. Change is inevitable. Survivors know how to evolve with the change. They dream new dreams and make with what they have and make something new and great. Adverse situations shake us up in our comfort zones, and we are compelled to think in innovative ways. As a result, we reinvent ourselves and rebuild lives.

Coronavirus has left us with two choices: give up or reinvent ourselves. Now you know you must choose the latter. Do you love yourself? Do you believe you deserve to be happy on this earth? Do you want to give your best to your loved ones? Then you have to find new ways and believe there is a life after the pandemic.

"It is easy to say," you think, "But how do I move forward from here?"

Your doubts are true. With what we have lost in this pandemic, it is hard to fathom how to move forward from here. But also know that your belief system is more powerful than you think it is. If you know how to convince your mind to achieve something, you will find ways to achieve it, no matter how difficult it may seem. But to achieve such a result, you need to be in a specific mindset. You need to understand that there is no magic, and yet the magic is in what you do and how you do it. There are two elements of Doing; they are Physical and Mental. If you build your Mental state to an Achiever's mind-set, the Physical work will take place in due course. Hence, it is most important that we start thinking about getting into the right way of thinking, into an Achiever's mind-set during the pandemic so at the end of 2021, we can come out with something solid, something we can look forward to.

We shall look into Mike Pegg's tools, the British confidence-building guru who has been improving mindsets for fifty years, and we shall think about how we can self-reflect and explore what else we can do and how we can prepare ourselves to achieve things.

Mike Pegg has been improving lives by building inner strengths and working on the consequences of weaknesses and how to overcome them. Mike ran a pioneering therapeutic community for young people in the 80s, and his work was featured in the BBC documentary "Escape to Fulfilment" in 1972. Mike set up his company in 1974 and has been helping people to achieve success ever since. Mike has written several books, including "The Positive Encourager's Book," a self-help guide that is inspirational and full of tips and tools helping to work towards a target.

Mike's guide has never been more helpful as it is in the current circumstances; therefore, let's look at how we can help ourselves from the growing frustration, worries, hopelessness many of us are suffering from during the pandemic. We shall use Mike's tools and guides and examine our everyday thoughts and beliefs and explore if it is at all possible to find new ways and build a life after the pandemic.

Mike tells us that if people focus on what they **believe** in, they can eventually achieve what they **believe.** The things we believe in deep down inside, the visions we have of the world, are the things we genuinely love. Imagine if those inner visions come true! How amazing would that be? Mike calls it "**Building Something Brilliant.**" Because what you love, when achieved, is what is **brilliant** to you.

Now you may argue that you are just an ordinary person, you just want to be happy and look after yourself and your family, that you have a small dream. You are not after anything brilliant. So many times have I witnessed people panicking when they mentioned that they could achieve something brilliant. This is because we imagine that **Brilliant** is something larger than life achievement like climbing Mount Everest or forming a multi-millionaire company. Yes, th**ese** things are brilliant too but remember that it is about you and you only. What is exciting and desired in your imagination is **Brilliant** in your world. The adrenaline and the satisfaction you will experience when you will bring your inner dreams into reality is actually the same as the climber who has achieved to see the peak of the Himalayans; because our dreams may be different, but the joy of success we experience is the same.

So, for example, perhaps you have always wanted to open a little shop selling specialty food from your grandparent's birth country. Why? Because you really believe this particular food has to be introduced to society because they have unique qualities and they shouldn't be forgotten. This is your inner desire, your vision of the world where

PSYCHOLOGY

people appreciate a dying art, and in your own way, this is how you have always felt you could help the community. Perhaps you have been doing the same job for many years, and you became comfortable. You never really enjoyed the job, but it offered you security, and you thought of your inner vision of having a specialty food store, connecting with people in a niche market, and helping the specialty producers was an unrealistic dream. Perhaps you are bounded by cultural identities and feel that although this is all you ever wanted to do, it is not a suitable occupation for you from a societal perspective.

However, the pandemic has confiscated your comfort, you don't have job security anymore, and you don't know what will happen after the pandemic. Think about it now, would it be so defiant to wanting to be the person you always wanted to be? To be brave enough to do what you want to isn't the most amazing and humble thing to do? And once you achieve it, imagine, from a societal perspective. It is you who will be the achiever because you have built something brilliant by making your dream come true.

Mike tells us that to build something **brilliant**, you need three elements.

Beliefs: You have to believe that you can achieve it, providing that you are fully committed to doing your very best to achieve your goals. Your motivational leader can make you believe that you can achieve something temporarily; however, if you don't have the faith developing from within, this belief will soon wither away. Hence, you need to work on your belief first. What is stopping you from not believing that you can't do something new?

You can write down your goal and then think of all the scenarios and possibilities. Make a realistic note on what you think is possible to achieve and what are maybe achievable. Now you have an idea of what things you can be sure about. Then think about what the things are you need help with; can it be possible with the help of a team or organisations, and what can you do to reach these people? Lastly, think about what is not practically possible in the current circumstances and how you can work around it. For example, you know that you cannot import a food item overnight in a pandemic, although a prompt service would make you stand out. In such a case, what will you do? Can you make this item in the home country? Can you cross this item out?

Basics: You have focused on what you can achieve, now, diligently, keep doing the basics required to achieve this goal. You will not achieve your goal if you take intervals in doing the basics because you felt tired or lost your belief momentarily. Yes, cynicism will grasp your internal state, and you may physically feel lethargic because of the negative thoughts; however, you still have to carry on with the basics even if you have to trudge along for a while. So the key is to keep looking after your health and mind because to carry on with basics, you need to stay positive. Therefore, adapt to a healthy lifestyle; follow a routine, turn up to the meetings, classes, and work schedules you are expected to on time. Blank out the negative speeches; people will indeed say some dispiriting things. It is not because people want you to fail. It is because people are scared, and they feel they are helping you by discouraging you. Have sympathy but do not nurture negative discourses. Now stay calm, do one thing at a time. Do not overstress yourself by making a hectic schedule; do a little at a time. The aim is to slowly gain control over yourself and your target. This will be a natural process, as you will slowly develop yourself, you will learn new things on this journey, and you will meet like-minded people who will guide you. You will learn how to overcome setbacks, you will keep improving yourself by knowing your weaknesses and strengths, but this can happen naturally only if you keep doing your best.

Brilliance: A great achiever or a great team keeps doing the basics and keeps building, and when appropriate, they add the brilliance. To achieve brilliance, you have to focus on your strengths rather than your weakness. You will build based on what you have got rather than what you haven't got. You will utilise what is available instead of focusing on what elements you need but don't have.

There is a great potential of losing hope or discouraging people by focusing on what they don't have. Although, this "I don't have" or "she/he doesn't have" is not a true situation. Let us try to understand it better.

Whether we want it or not, our society is full of diverse people. We can be dyslexic, be in a wheelchair, might be highly sensitive, and have depression and anxiety, perhaps have autism or a physical illness. Then some are over-enthusiastic, amazing in a particular thing but get bored with the rest of the responsibilities easily. We have different neurological make-up, and we process information differently. Few are late developers, and others tend to move way ahead, leaving the peers behind.

It is important that we don't see these as obstacles and the reasons for us to be non-achievers by default. Instead of thinking these qualities are a problem to build a meaningful life, they can be seen as a part of the make-up of a person who would enable them to be what they need to be. Albert Einstein, the most influential German Physicist of the twentieth century, was dyslexic. In school, he loved science and maths, but he disliked grammar and always had problems with spelling. His teachers declared him as a borderline intellectually impaired child. Can we state that it is his dyslexia that enabled him to focus on science only? It surely makes sense if we understand that we are here with certain traits, and these traits sometimes overtake other qualities, and perhaps this basic make-up is needed to make us what we are, in what we achieve brilliance in. Einstein later said,

"Everybody is a genius. But if you judge a fish by its **ability** to climb a tree, it will live its whole life believing that it is stupid."

If you keep comparing yourself with someone who has something in their basic make-up instead of what you have in your make-up, you will not be able to continue with the **basics** and add **brilliance** to it.

Next, Mike tells us about the **Driven approach**. Great achievers are focused on a certain path; they follow a chosen discipline and can often be daring. They confront disappointments and achievements on the way; they deal with the drama and do not get destructed by their surroundings. Their ultimate focuses are to learn, achieve, acquire, and deliver. The Australian American motivational speaker Nick Vujicic was born without limbs. He is the star of the short film "The Butterfly Circus" and the founder of "Life without limbs" and a writer of several books on how to surpass the negativity around us and outshine in a chosen principle. Therefore, it will be a great challenge for us to re-build ourselves without the **driven approach**.

Start constructing a visual image of what can be achieved at the end of the road? Start thinking about what drives you. Perhaps:

You want to provide care to the elderly.

You want to provide for your family.

You want to achieve a certain qualification.

You want to take care of animals.

What drives you is based on who you are, your make-up, on how you want to see the world, and there is no right and wrong or what is acceptable or not acceptable. To give you an example, I once attended a global conference for women who have achieved excellence. I met a lady from the Middle-East who received national recognition for developing the state-of-the-art sewerage system. She told us that she was always interested in the drainage system and wanted to develop it since she was a child. People around her would tease her by blocking their nose when she was hired in the city sewage department. She was determined that she was going to improve city life, and within a few years, with her driven approach, she not only achieved her goal but gained recognition from the public, which means that when she started

PSYCHOLOGY

working, it wasn't socially acceptable for a woman of her high status to work for the drainage department, but she was not fazed by the drama around her. Hence an ability to overlook the standard social concepts of what is normality or what is acceptable or possible is required.

An achiever will think about their dreams and aims before they will commit. This is a part of the Decision-Making ability you have to focus on. Explore the potential way forward and consider the possible implications. This is done differently by different people. Some people work through this logically, and some people make prompt decisions. With decision making, Mike tells us that the following may be useful:

- To clarify the real results, you want to achieve and translate this into a clear picture of success;
- To clarify the key strategies, you can follow to achieve the picture of success;
- To clarify the pluses and minuses involved in working to achieve the picture of success.

Remember that to be the achiever and making your dreams into reality, you have to embark with your eyes open. It will help you to check on your motivation and commitments. You will be able to consider the pluses and minuses in achieving your goal; you will have a realistic outlook.

"…Those who dream by night may or may not follow up… Dreamers of the day are dangerous … for they may act their dreams with open eyes, to make it possible" T E Lawrence (British archaeologist, army officer, and Writer).

Discipline is a quality-asset of an achiever. Great achievers take delight in following certain disciplines. They follow a rhythm and do the right thing in the right way. They may use the following steps:

- They explore the real results they want to achieve and clarify their destination.
- They clarify the steps they can take – the principles to follow and the practical tasks to be done – to reach their destination.
- They focus on doing each of these things properly on the way towards reaching their destination.

Once you can adapt to a life of discipline to achieve your goal, you can think of:

- How can I keep developing?
- How can I build a repertoire or become invaluable to the organisation?
- How can I tackle the areas of improvements?
- How can I apply this knowledge to deliver great results?

You have now chosen your path and found your discipline. So now it is time to be Daring. By looking at how far you have come now, you may decide that you have more to gain and less to lose if you dream in the daylight and follow it calculatively. Therefore, this is what you get:

Discipline => Daring => Desired Results

As a great achiever, you will know that sometimes you will return home feeling down, and in counterpart, some nights will be full of great feelings. You can accept this reality before it has started to happen and begin keeping a log of the experience. You may reflect on the delights and disappointments and think about how you could improve the beaten issues.

Dealing with dramas

We have already discussed that as a great achiever, you will not focus on the drama on your journey. Do not get sidetracked by individuals who choose to be dramatic, negative, seeing problems instead of solutions. Think about How:

- Can I prevent these dramas from happening? How can I deal with any dramas if, despite my best efforts, they do happen?
- Can I buy time to think? How can I focus on the real results to achieve in the short-term and long-term? How can I do my best to find possible solutions to the dramas? How can I implement these solutions?
- Can I return to following the required disciplines? How can I get a quick success? How can I continue doing good work on the way towards the destination?

You will find your rhythm back once you have worked out the above.

Delivery

Whatever day-dream you have decided to pursue, say you want to be an entrepreneur, an artist, a writer, a professional; you have to ultimately deliver. Great workers often go into a relaxed relentlessness mode. Meaning that you need to continue your basics and add your brilliance at a relaxed pace, but you have to be at it relentlessly. You may want to separate the relaxed and relentless modes into two elements but remember that you need to take care of yourself in this journey. It is better if you know how to pursue your dream relentlessly but in a stride that you can control, that you are doing it at a relaxed pace. This is where self-care comes, such as a variety of relaxation therapy, meditation, a routine between life and work, listening to music, or spending time with your loved ones.

This is a good time to explore if something else to be done if you need to change the gear to achieve the target. We may start our journey with something specific in mind, but things may change on the way. In such circumstances, we cannot give up and get back to where we were before, but we can think about new paths and ask for different types of help; because we know we are still going towards the same goal. So when the negative thought comes into the mind because something on the way has changed, close your eyes, and start visualizing the end of this journey and re-instate your belief.

To find out how Hypnotherapy can help to achieve the relaxed and relentless approach towards achieving goals, visit https://hypnosis.plus/.

Your feedback on this article

I really loved your writing. The article is excellent, simple n easy, more important it gives a thought about my life how I have been overcoming many struggles in my mind which were affecting my physical self.

Rosy Fernandez; Sales Consultant (UK)

What you wrote is so brilliant and so true, a lot of will people think and most will be able to connect with what was written and what most are thinking as well; it was like you were in many others mind, I think and say the same to others and in health and wellbeing, being supportive of each other and working with each other's strengths, there is so much more to be said in part 2, 3, 4, etc., would be very welcomed.

Sal; Volunteer at Health & Wellbeing Group (UK)

HYPNOTHERAPY

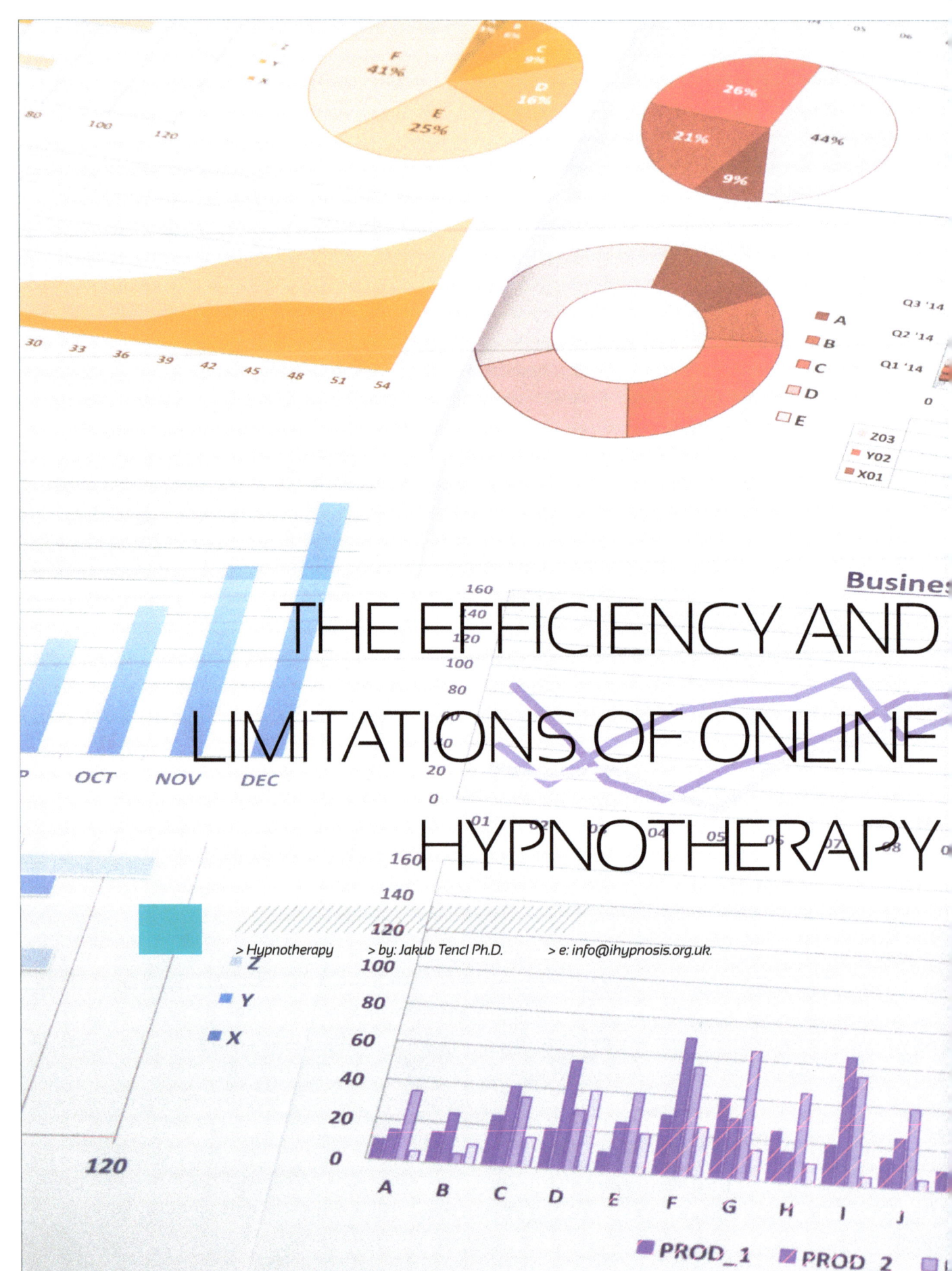

THE EFFICIENCY AND LIMITATIONS OF ONLINE HYPNOTHERAPY

> Hypnotherapy   > by: Jakub Tencl Ph.D.   > e: info@ihypnosis.org.uk.

HYPNOTHERAPY

Abstract

The effectiveness of online hypnotherapy is currently not quite clear, therefore in 2020 a survey collecting statistical data about common cases performed online was conducted and the collected data may serve for further exploration. Furthermore, as an outcome of observation, a type of personality that may reap the most benefit and what areas are suitable for online hypnotherapy had to be proposed.

Hypnosis, the main tool in hypnotherapy, suggests creating a perceptive conscious mind. Hypnotherapy online may have technical and psychological limitations. Some associations even discourage performing induction online. It will therefore be useful to determine the criteria for online hypnotherapy, and the criteria will need further discussion. The goal is not to reject the option of hypnotherapy online, but to find a solution that will be most effective in terms of circumstances.

Introduction

The survey was conducted from the second half of 2020 to the first half of 2021. 11 hypnotherapists completed the anonymous survey. Members of The National Hypnotherapy Society and The British Association of Therapists and Hypnotherapists were approached. Questions regarded the period from March to October 2020 during which restrictions were mandatory due to COVID-19. Not all questions were answered for unknown reasons. Let's assume that statistics of the cases in the practice of hypnotherapy are generally not considered important, therefore, professional associations in the field should have mechanisms to collect such data in order to direct development. Another assumption is that the number of cases significantly decreased during the mentioned period.

It is obvious that a survey with a low number of respondents may be inconclusive. Nevertheless, the following survey may show:

- tendencies influenced by the pandemic
- effectiveness in terms of the number of successfully closed cases
- the proportion of successful face-to-face and online meetings
- the proportion of specific goals and their success which can determine the area most suitable for online hypnotherapy
- the self-confidence of hypnotherapists to perform hypnotherapy online which may imply further training
- technological prowess.

Results

Difficulties during performed sessions (9 respondents, assuming the rest do not have a problem)

77.8%	Poor internet connection
11.1%	Insufficient knowledge of work with clients online
33.3%	Concern about unforeseen events during the session
22.2%	The client fell asleep
33.3%	Clients generally do not have confidence in sessions online

20% of respondents do not feel confident to work with clients online while 80% do (10 respondents, 1 respondent did not answer the question, which might mean that s/he had not had hypnotherapy online).

30% of respondents feel the need for support in work via online platforms while 70% do not (10 respondents, 1 respondent did not answer).

Interpretation

The biggest issue is the internet connection; therefore, it might be useful to have at least two internet connections. The other pointers show that training in how to perform hypnotherapy online might be needed. In case of concerns about unforeseen events, it is suggested not to perform hypnotherapy online. In terms of clients who fell asleep, it is suggested to change the approach in the initial evaluation or the intervention of a supervisor. The initial evaluation of clients can include examining the criteria described in this paper. The goal is to (naturally) prevent sleep during the next session. Once a client is sleeping, it is recommended to choose a considerate way of waking him/her up.

The number of clients from March to October 2020 (10 respondents, 1 respondent did not answer).

0 - 10	40%
11 - 30	50%
More than 101	10%

Interpretation

It seems that the average was between 11 and 30 clients. We don't have statistical data to compare with other periods, but the low number in this range implies 11 clients seen weekly, which means 44 sessions monthly. Did the influence of the COVID-19 pandemic decrease or increase the number of clients? Assuming that the trend of active online communication has become dominant once there was no other way due to the restrictions, it is reasonable to expect that the demand for hypnotherapy online will increase. But it is inconclusive since there are no other data for comparison.

The number of clients who underwent hypnotherapy online (10 respondents, 1 respondent did not answer).

Stopping smoking	100%	0-10 clients
Weight loss and management	70%	0-10 clients
	30%	11-30 clients
Stress management	70%	0-10 clients
	20%	11-30 clients
	10%	31-50 clients
Phobias	100%	0-10 clients
Anxiety	60%	0-10 clients
	30%	11-30 clients
	10%	31-50 clients

Interpretation

There may seem to be comorbidities that may be interpreted as the clients seeking to become nonsmokers may feel a need to get slimmer, but at the same time, the need for managing stress can automatically arise as part of the treatment. Anxiety might be involved too. Phobias might be isolated or related to stress and anxiety. The results show that phobias and smoking figure to 100% in 0-10 clients in a defined period. Unless it is capnophobia, there may be a misleading understanding that smoking relates to phobias.

The success of online hypnotherapy (10 respondents)

50%	0-10 cases
40%	11-30 cases
10%	81-100 cases

The success rate in online hypnotherapy

In terms of the number of clients, we can calculate the range between lower and higher success rates.

We have on average range from 5 to 50 clients and success in 5 to 90 cases on average. We will calculate an average from these ranges $((5+50)/2) + ((5+90)/2)/2 = $ **37.5** which can be considered as the **coefficient of the success** and in the percentage 27.5 of 47.5 is a **57.9% success rate.**

Due to the low number of respondents, we can conclude that this number is a guideline, and further surveys are needed.

The number of cases for ordinary goals that are divided into online and face-to-face hypnotherapy (8 respondents; this suggests lack of statistical data or that the cases were only online)

Stopping smoking	87.5%	0-10 cases
	12.5%	11-30 cases
Weight loss and management	100%	0-10 cases

HYPNOTHERAPY

Stress management	87.5%	0-10 cases
	12.5%	11-30 cases
Anxiety	75%	0-10 cases
	25%	11-30 cases
Phobias	87.5%	0-10 cases
	12.5%	11-30 cases

Interpretation

You can see that 0-10 cases are recorded on average and the only 100% result was weight loss and management which can be considered to be in high demand in hypnotherapeutic intervention.

Unsuccessful cases performed only online (7 respondents; this suggests that the rest were successful or inconclusive)

100%   0-10 cases

Unsuccessful cases performed partly online and in-person (8 respondents; this suggests that the rest were successful or inconclusive)

100%   0-10 cases

The rate of unsuccessful cases

In terms of the number of clients, we can deduce the average rate of unsuccessful cases.

We have on average range from 5 to 50 clients and 5 unsuccessful cases on average. So the formula will use an average from the range of the number of clients: $(((5+50)/2) + 5)/2 = 16.25$ which can be considered as the **coefficient of unsuccessful cases** and in percentage 5 of 27.5 = **18.2%** which is **the rate of unsuccessful cases**.

These numbers are valid based on results for hypnotherapy only online or divided into online and in person.

The personality suitable for online hypnotherapy

The suitable profile is not stated based on evidence, but observation in private hypnotherapy practice during 2020.

So far it is possible to propose the following criteria:

- Dissociative states of mind are not suitable for online hypnotherapy.
- The type of associated preference should be auditory.
- The number of online sessions should be limited even though the case is not closed. The total number of sessions is dependent on the type of the case. The need to interrupt treatment may arise from dynamic nonverbal signals verified at least in two consecutive sessions.
- Personality traits should be extroverted. They are for instance:
  - Enjoy social settings
  - Don't like or need a lot of time alone
  - Thrive on being around people
  - Friends with many people
  - Prefer to talk about problems or questions
  - Outgoing and optimistic.

List of diagnoses specified in ICD-11 that may be suitable for online hypnotherapy

6B00	Generalised anxiety disorder
6B02	Agoraphobia
6B04	Social anxiety disorder
6B0Y	Other specified anxiety or fear-related disorders
6E40.1	Psychological symptoms affecting disorders or diseases classified elsewhere
6E40.2	Personality traits or coping style affecting disorders or diseases classified elsewhere
6E40.4	Stress-related physiological response affecting disorders or diseases classified elsewhere

It is suggested to choose CBT for further diagnosed conditions in which spoken therapy can be performed online and hypnosis in person. However, goals characterized for hypnotherapy that are not stated in ICD-11 such as smoking and weight loss and management can be performed online, but initial evaluation should show possible comorbidities that will need a medical referral or session in person. The initial consultation therefore shows whether online or in-person is the most suitable form in the frame of the treatment plan.

Conclusion

Although this paper describes the need to determine limitations in online hypnotherapy and its success rate and rate of unsuccessful cases, there is room for discussion and further research.

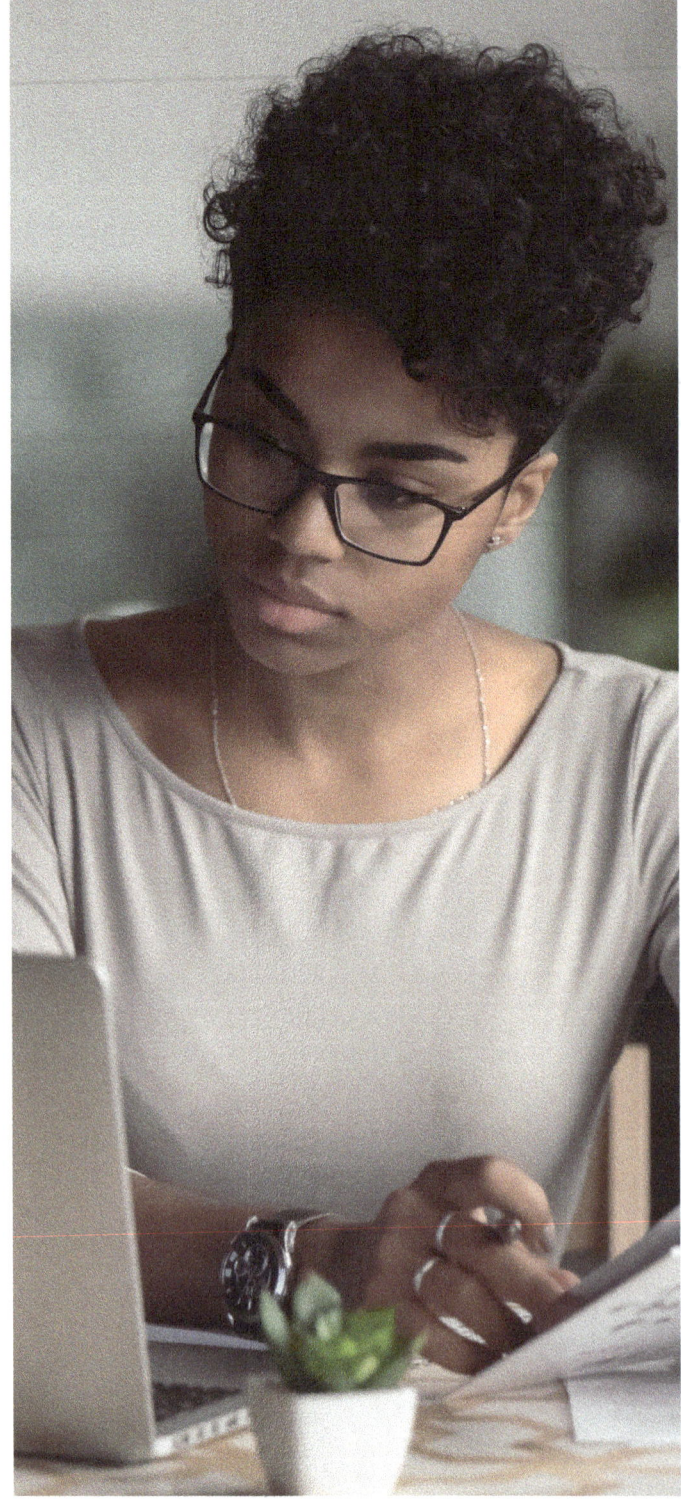

SERVICES AT HYPNOSIS PLUS

Here is the price list of services:

Press Release: £12*

Press Release with an interview, combo:

£60 publishing
£20 we will write a press release

Promotional article or interviews: £50.00*

Unrelated promotional articles: non-refundable one-off fee £500.00*

Promotional videos (short length: press release or introductory video): £50**

Product and service ads: £50 or £25 monthly***

Product and services video ads: £50**

Job Vacancy ad/Student recruitment ads: £15****

iHypnosis TV recording: £50 or £25 monthly**

IHypnosis TV feature-length interviews, educational or introductory videos or talks: £200*****

iHypnosis TV-placing ads: £50 or £25 monthly**

iHypnosis Radio-placing ads: £20 + £15 for an ad****

Hypnosis Radio-placings talks, interviews: £100

Requests for publishing own articles: £20

* The article has to be provided to fulfil the service.
** A video has to be provided to fulfil the service.
*** An ad has to be provided to fulfil the service.
**** The text has to be provided to fulfil this service.
***** A personal meeting in London for recording is necessary.

Upon request is possible to assist with video or graphic artwork, based on requirements will be stated the price afterwards.

In case of your interest please send an email at info@hypnosis.plus

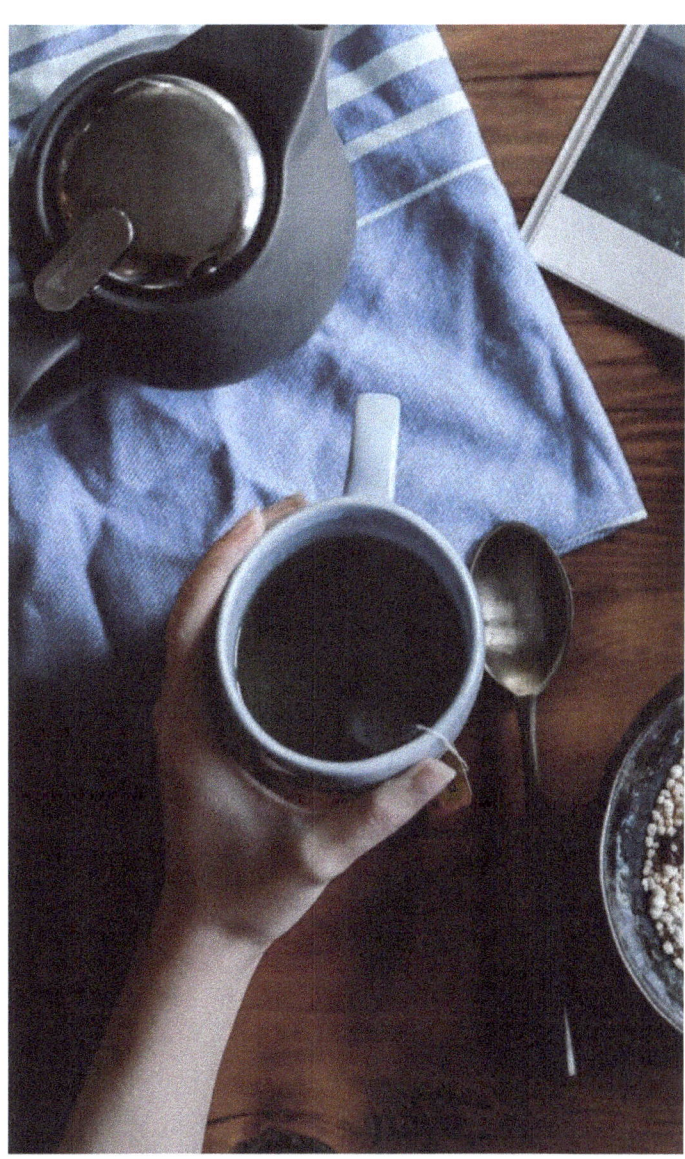

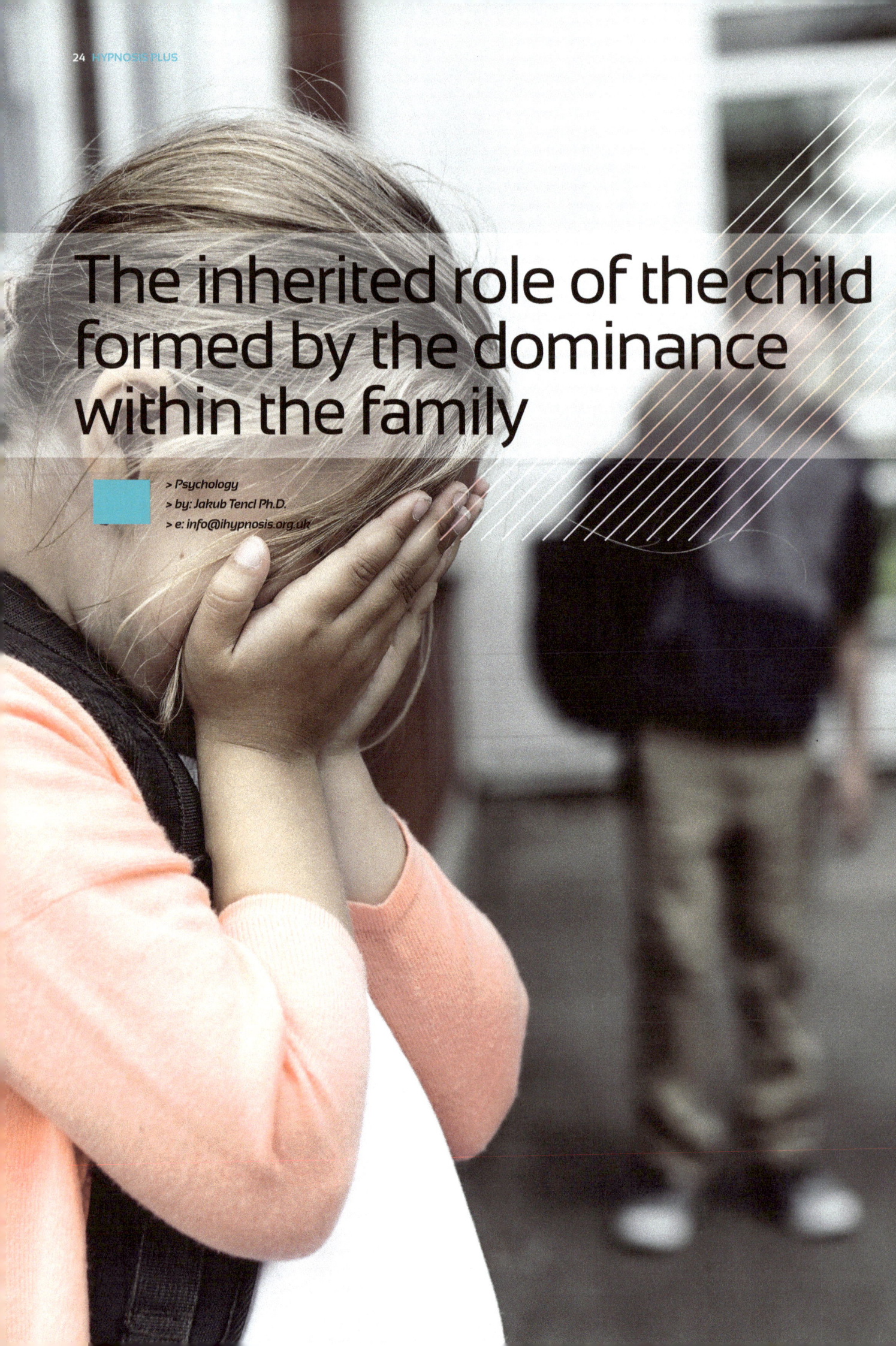

The inherited role of the child formed by the dominance within the family

> Psychology
> by: Jakub Tencl Ph.D.
> e: info@ihypnosis.org.uk

PSYCHOLOGY

Let's think about what may determine whether a child becomes a bully or will be bullied. The goal is to identify the relationships and personality characteristics in family dynamics and how they relate to each other.

The Karpman drama triangle describes the role of rescuer, victim, and persecutor where all roles are switched according to what the situation calls for. The roles do not have functional relationships, therefore individuals can be led to seeking substitute solutions outside the family environment.

Children develop, therefore inherit their roles inspired by interactions in the family.

If that is true, we need to focus firstly on how parents influence each other. Is the relationship balanced or are there hints of dominance? If yes, what role does the child inherit?

Here is what the schema looks like. The child usually learns from the mother how to perceive and from the father how to behave - interact with the outer world. The preference of learning from the same gender in certain aspects can play a role. However, in a scenario where the father shows dominance in interaction with the mother the child can inherit the role of the persecutor which he or she will apply outside the family environment, for instance at school. Hence it is the role of a bully. The child learns how to apply dominance. This is because the child learns interaction with the outer world from the father. Let's call it **axiom A**. The question is whether this is valid either for boys and girls or only for boys. I lean more towards the idea that this axiom applies more to boys considering the mentioned preference. In a scenario where the described interaction is perceived by girls, there may be the more inherited role of being bullied. However, when the girl needs it, she can have the attitude of the persecutor. Let's call this scenario **axiom A 1**.

What happens when there is dominance on the mother's side? The role of being bullied outside the family environment can develop. The child may have difficulty developing defence mechanisms because there is no learning of them in the development of perception if we follow the idea that the mother is the source of learning how to perceive and the father is the source of learning how to interact with the outer world. This may influence boys and girls alike. Let's call this scenario **axiom B**.

Dominance on the mother's side can determine the type of personality. Here we could distinguish according to Dr. Kappas between "emotional" or "physical" sexuality (defines the type of behaviour) and suggestibility. In this scenario, the dominant mother belongs to physical sexuality and the father belongs to emotional sexuality. Let's call this **criterion A**.

When dominance is on the father's side, it's the other way around. The father is more physically and the mother more emotionally sexual. Let's call this **criterion B**.

Here the question arises whether sexual behaviours are developed based on the relationship dynamic, therefore it could be misleading. Let's suppose that this is a rare case.

We need to describe a scenario when dominance is on both sides. This probably never happens at an equal level, if so, the family may break up. And the type of personality in this scenario will be inconclusive. On the outer level, it may look to be 50% emotional and 50% physical sexuality. Let's consider this to be **axiom C**.

Now the question is how the child will act towards each parent in the described scenarios. That could also reinforce the chosen role outside the family environment.

In the case of axiom A, the mother's dominance will be presented to the child and have a direct or indirect influence. And the child will have the need to influence the mother. The father's influence is in a sense a defence, thus unwanted manipulation. The child will therefore not develop the ability to defend himself, so may be bullied outside the family environment. The child can develop a perception of distorted reality due to chronic emotional suppression. Thus there may be a dissociation which can at a manageable level serve as reinforcement of emotional patterns.

In the case of axiom B, the child attempts to influence both parents, though the father's dominance will have a direct or indirect influence. Consistency of the father's dominance can reinforce the child acting as a persecutor outside the family environment. In case of inconsistency of the father's dominance, the child will attempt to take over the role of persecutor and try to create more consistency in his dominance.

In the case of axiom C, it is more likely that the child may be completely dissociated, disconnected, and there will be no successful attempts in any kind of influence from the parents' side. The reason may be that due to balanced emotional and physical sexuality the child will be able to adapt as required.

It may be worth briefly discussing suggestibility based on the previous context. Considering that the child is developing its suggestibility, we can talk about the parents. Emotional suggestibility suggests the attitude of defence and physical suggestibility suggests the attitude of dominance. That would describe the intention of emotional or physical sexuality in behaviour.

When parents have balanced emotional and physical sexuality, the determination of suggestibility due to the ability to adapt is not clear.

Emotional sexuality and suggestibility

A type of sexual behaviour in which the individual reacts with defensive emotions to prevent his/her physical body from feeling, thereby exaggerating emotional needs. EMOTIONAL SUGGESTIBILITY – suggestible behaviour characterized by a high degree of responsiveness to inferred suggestions affecting the emotions, and a restriction of responses of the physical body, usually associated with hypnoidal depth.

Physical sexuality and suggestibility

Sexual behaviour in which the individual reacts to physical stimulation as a defence to protect his/her emotional behaviour, thereby exaggerating the need for physical acceptance and gratification. PHYSICAL SUGGESTIBILITY - suggestible behaviour characterized by a high degree of responsiveness to suggestions affecting the body and a restriction of emotional responses, usually associated with cataleptic stages or deeper.

The Karpman drama triangle

The Karpman drama triangle is a social model of human interaction proposed by Stephen B. Karpman. The triangle maps a type of destructive interaction that can occur among people in conflict.

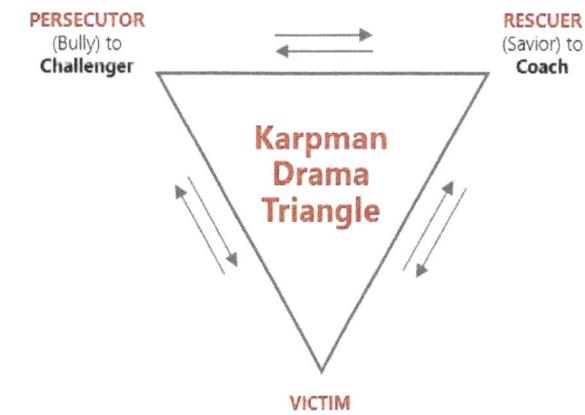

HYPNOTHERAPY

> Hypnotherapy
> by: Shanta Sultana
> e; shanta.sultana@hypnosis.plus

WHY RESEARCH OF CLINICAL HYPNOTHERAPY MUST FLOURISH

Interview with Mr Peter Mabbutt, the President of the British Society of Clinical Hypnosis (BSCH)

"Hypnotherapy must be doing something right because it keeps coming back into the medical field. My message to the drug companies is if you invest, we shall do the research on hypnotherapy for you, and eventually, it will bring the profit to you," says Mr Peter Mabbutt, the President of the British Society of Clinical Hypnosis (BSCH) and the Head of Academics at London School of Clinical Communication and Hypnosis (LSCCH).

Recent experiences including LSCCH studies show that clinical hypnotherapy has played a significant role during the pandemic in a variety of sectors including caring for the healthcare professions. Clinical Hypnotherapy continues to assist a diverse range of mental and physical ailments and yet, there is a tendency of pushing it aside and debating over its proven validity. Why is this so and who is dismissing it? How can we bring the understanding of the mind and body connection to the general public?

Peter Mabbutt, with his extensive research background in the field, answers some of the pivotal questions on the present and future of the research of Hypnotherapy to Hypnosis Plus; essential "know-how" for the students and practitioners of Clinical Hypnotherapy.

Can you tell us something about your background as a researcher?

I was originally trained as a psychopharmacologist. I was at Guys & Thomas's working on anxiety, phobias, and also worked on depression and panic attacks. But those days, the emphasis was on drug treatment instead of psychotherapeutic treatment. I decided to make a career change and trained as a hypnotherapist. I became involved with a project with the Guy's & Thomas's hospital called, "The Health Education & Lifestyle Therapy for Hyper-Tension Programme," where we were working with hypertensive patients. I was offering stress management and relaxation in the form of hypnosis, and the colleagues were teaching them physical exercises and providing nutritional advice and other healthy lifestyle advice. One of the areas I was involved in there was pain management. We started working with the University of Malaya where Brachial Plexus[1] Injury is a common occurrence. The pain generated by this injury is notorious and challenging to manage pharmacologically. They wanted us to apply hypnotherapy to manage it, and we had some good results. Patients suffering from pain were finally able to sleep. Others were able to return to work, and from there the "Hypnotherapy Pain Unit" was developed.

Back in the U.K., we also did a research project on cardiac patients and we wanted to see if hypnotherapy could help to protect the post-infarct heart and the study indicated that it certainly helped to cope with the stress better.

What is "psychoneuroimmunology"? Tell us something about the research on the mind and body connection. In psychoneuroimmunology, where does hypnotherapy stand? What studies are available?

Psychoneuroimmunology is about the connection between the mind and body; this concept has been around a long time that the mind and the immune system are inextricably linked. Cartesian Dualist[2] idea convinced us for a long time that the mind and body are completely separate entities. However, recent scientific researches have proven that the mind and body are very much linked which also means that the mind and the disease state are also very much linked. It doesn't mean you can think yourself to disease but the mindset and the emotion you apply to approach the disease have an impact on the immune system. We now know that the immune system is partly involved in the production of many of our moods, i.e. depression and anxiety, and we also know that our nervous system is involved with our immunology which is our immune system protecting the body.

In a balanced body and balanced mind, everything is working in its optimal state but if you tip into a disease state, it is accompanied by a negative mindset. Researches show that the outcomes are poorer with a negative mindset primarily because of the mind and body connection. The immune system is using the time moderating and modulating the negative emotions instead of following its main purpose that is to manage the body's ability to heal. The mind-body connection is all about recognizing and understanding this and then having the ability to use forms of therapy to improve mindsets, bringing the sense of coping, sense of happiness, sense of pleasure. It doesn't mean you will go on celebrating a disease such as cancer. It is not like, "Great I have cancer," but more like, "I accept I have cancer. This is the reality, and I shall do everything within my abilities with a positive attitude to cope well with it." The idea is that the positive mindset gets the immune system doing what it is supposed to do.

Think about the many factors involved in developing tumours. One factor is called Tumour Necrosis Factor-alpha, or TNF Alpha, and with TNF Alpha we are thinking tumour, cancer, necrosis, killing. This is what it does along with various other things. However, we also know that TNF Alpha is modulating our stress response. The human body is designed to have both long and short-term survival priorities. Our stress response is on the fight-flight response, and it is our response to depredation. When the Sabre-Tooth tiger jumped in front of the cave person, the fight-flight response kicked in which meant we had a choice of fighting or running away to survive. Now if you look at traumatized animals, they seek refuge in a corner or their nests and they become quiet. That's what the early humans did and had a better response to stress than we modern humans do. They would return to their caves or villages, lay down, and rest, hence the stress responses would switch off. So immediate survival priority was pushing everything into "let's help you live by running away."

In modern days, when we go into a stress response, i.e. Covid stress which plays a variety of pressures on us, our fight-flight response kicks in but it stays on and on. The longer it does that the least time the TNF Alpha works; for example, this opens up the opportunity for the cancer cells to divide and start forming the tumour. I remember a wonderful phrase: "The prolonged stress turns TNF Alpha to the dark side and becomes a cancer promoter." The good news is, if you take the stress away it rebalances the system. Stress response impacts heavily on our immune system which is why stressed people get ill rapidly and also negative emotions generate a poorer outcome with long-term diseases compared to the people with long-term diseases with a positive

HYPNOTHERAPY

emotional state.

There are many studies out there looking at the mind and body connection and how hypnotherapy can be used to improve mood and the sense of coping. There is a whole pantheon of approaches that one can apply; it is about helping people and about a positive mindset, changing condition responses; I.e. when one hears the word cancer, instead of having a shocking reaction one can have a calm and positive acceptance meaning that instead of giving up they have a mind-set to follow all they were told to do. Hypnotherapy can program a person to help have these positive responses but also remember that the very act of going under hypnosis has a positive impact on the body and immune system.

Studies have shown that when someone goes under hypnosis for pro-Inflammatory Cytokines[3], these things are reduced in the body so that's a good thing. Looking at covid disease, a lot of pro-Inflammatory Cytokines are released in the body during covid, and it is not meant to say that hypnosis would heal covid but perhaps hypnosis can help to bring the level of inflammation down. We know that there are types of depression that haven't been quantified yet that show increasing the level of pro-Inflammatory Cytokines. Hypnosis on these researches showed that it was reducing the inflammation level although it wasn't its primary intention. Current researches show that one of the best approaches is combining hypnosis with cognitive-behavioural therapy (CBT) for depression; it is effective on a psychological level but also effective on the physiological state.

If you think about being guided into a hypnotic state, you are turning on the parasympathetic nervous system, and you are moving into a resting and digestive state. In this state, you have muscular relaxation which is excellent for pain management, and there is the reduction of pro-Inflammatory Cytokines and also the heart hence the respiration starts to slow down significantly pulling the blood pressure down. So, hypertensive clients positively benefit just going into the hypnotic state. Researches have shown that hypnosis and any form of relaxation can permanently bring the blood pressure down, even when we don't know the cause of hypertension.

You have been influential in setting up a Pain Management clinic and pain research program at the University of Malaya. What kind of pain can be managed with hypnotherapy? Is there any research currently happening on pain management with hypnotherapy? If yes, what is the status?

Any pain can be managed with hypnotherapy. We have been examining applying hypnosis during surgery, i.e. carpal[4] tunnel surgery and brachial plexus surgery. As I have mentioned earlier, a large number of people are the victim of motorbike and moped crashes in Malaysia that snaps the collarbone. The brachial plexus is underneath the collarbone where lots of different nerves are coming together and breaking that causes intense pain. I have already mentioned that it is extremely difficult to manage with pharmacological remedies and so hypnosis comes in here. Hypnosis can manage the cancer pain of all stages and other pain people suffer from at the end of life timescale. There are very good researches proving that hypnosis can help burn victims into a guided imagery state which helps to manage pain but it also helps to reduce the stress hormone of the flight-fight response and reduces the blistering improving healing rates. This positive effect has been seen in bone fracture-related injuries as well. Virtually all pain can be managed with hypnotherapy, however, we have to understand that people have to be willing to go under the hypnotic procedure.

I had a very bad leg injury with torn muscles and badly damaged tendons, and it was painful. With self-hypnosis, I converted the feeling of pain to a sensation of pressure. This showed me that something was wrong with my body, and I need to take care of it without having to suffer. I have used hypnotherapy in dental pain on myself and others, and one can go under dental operations and procedures without the help of an anaesthetic when under hypnotherapy. The interesting opinion is this is just a placebo effect but the brain scan studies have shown which areas of the brain are involved under the hypnotic treatment. When someone is pretending to be in a hypnotic state or under pharmacological treatment, these areas of the brain are not lit up in the scans. When I was working on my pain it was changing the nature of my pain in the somatosensory[5] cortex by converting the pain into pressure.

The anterior[6] cingulate cortex modulates the perception of suffering amongst a few other things that it does. Under hypnotic management, the anterior cingulate cortex area does not light up. So the scanning studies show us that these are not just placebo effects. Understanding neurochemistry further, the hypnotic suggestion influences serotonin, oxytocin, glutamate, and dopamine and is converted with the efficacy of hypnotic suggestion. Having gone through a denial stage of hypnotherapy, we are moving on to understanding more and more about it which is probably why the medical profession has started to take it seriously. Perhaps the last 10-20 years or more, the medical professionals have been supportive of hypnotherapy; British Medical Association (BMA) has been endorsing hypnotherapy since 1955 and the American Medical Association followed up in 1956; Indian Medical Association, Malaysian Medical Association has followed, and many other associations globally will be following; it is an interesting time.

What other research studies can you mention on the proven effect of hypnotherapy and are you participating in any of them?

The largest number of research is on pain management. There are proven records of helping to overcome a wide range of phobia and there is research on trauma. I am particularly interested in trauma and mind and body connection research. There are also skin-related problems such as eczema and psoriasis. The old saying is, "the skin is the mirror of our emotions." In the fetus, the skin develops from the same cells as the nervous system; due to this link, when people are stressed, they express it on the skin, on the t-zone of the face. Hypnotherapy helps to break that link and addresses underlying stress issues that might be contributing to the skin condition. Virtually anything that has an emotive component, hypnotherapy will be able to help with. Looking at psychosomatic illness, hypnotherapy is an excellent approach to understand what are the underlying emotional triggers. Hypnotherapy first uncovers what it is, then works through what it is, and lastly sets the client up with a future where they can avoid experiencing these pains and conditions.

At present, my research is focused on two levels. They are developing the courses at LSCCH and developing our international online therapy centre. Nevertheless, I am in the periphery of the research arena as people often consult me with questions, and I assist externally. I am not involved in any overt or face-to-face research at present.

In your opinion, are there not enough studies globally in hypnotherapy? What research in hypnotherapy is lacking and what more in your opinion can be done?

I think we are just scratching the surface in regards to the proven effect of hypnotherapy. We need to understand more about neurology. We need to know more about neurochemistry; neurology is becoming quite advanced but more understanding is required. Neurochemistry is not readily understood at present.

I also think the research should be integrated with conventional medicine; BMA stated that hypnotherapy is neither complementary nor an alternative method but it is an integrative treatment. I think we need a good number of advanced studies integrating hypnotherapy with conventional medicine. The proven effect of hypnotherapy will reduce the cost of medical treatment significantly. A patient can go under a treatment without sedatives and anaesthesia under hypnosis and after the procedure, the patient may not need a chaperon home because the client's body is chemical-free which also means the patient does not have to stay at the recovery unit. The patient will spend sufficient time to be checked if they are fit to perform however do not need an extensive period for the sedatives to wear away. All these reduce costs.

More research is needed on the post-use of hypnotherapy and how it affects the post-operative healing rates.

I don't know how hypnotherapy is applied to people who are having a heart attack but there is much literature based on anecdotal accounts on people surviving heart attacks under hypnotherapy in planes for example. How relaxation and going into a trance state can assist a cardiac attack should have research. Research in fracture healing is also needed as some accounts show that fracture healings were rapid under hypnotic treatments. There are many questions to answer and a vast amount of studies are needed. So it goes back to my early days in psychopharmacology and my interest in understanding neurochemistry and neurology.

What is the future of research in hypnotherapy and why is it important?

We need to open new avenues of treating people and new avenues of understanding the human body. One of the big questions I always had was in the early years when I was working with a group of drugs known as benzodiazepines[7] - the valiums of the world. We discovered that there are particular receptors in the brain for benzodiazepines; why has the brain got a receptor for drugs? So what was the substance that was binding these receptors and does this substance have anything to do with a hypnotic response? Benzodiazepines are referred to as sedative-hypnotic drugs because they mimic the state of hypnosis; Do these drugs make us drowsy because they are mimicking the substance that has something to do with the hypnotic response? Is it because they are binding to the receptors that are making us drowsy?

On whole, it is about understanding the human body and mind and understanding new ways of helping people in conjunction with modern medicine. I believe the current happenings will bring hypnotherapy more and more into the medical arena; if you think about it, it had a huge role to play before pharmacological practices taking over. Drugs came in and hypnotherapy and psychotherapy were shoved aside. People are again understanding they may have a stronger role to play globally. Also can't ignore the cost-effectiveness of hypnotherapy. Research on cost-effective hypnotherapeutic treatment will help to release the medical funds for other areas of treatments, so it is certainly something to be looked into.

In your opinion are there enough options and opportunities to conduct research in hypnotherapy? Any idea on how to increase the prospects and interest to conduct further research?

I think people like us who have the interest to talk about it; i.e. I give talks in the hospitals, in conferences- is a way to raise interests and opportunities. Hypnotherapy should be introduced via broadcast and print media. The problem is, where does the funding come from? I am not a conspiracy theorist, and I don't want to sound like one. But the reality is a lot of funding comes from drug companies. Hypnotherapy is not a drug, therefore the interest in funding hypnotherapy research is not there. There is some funding available out there but the challenge is to bring this research into universities and in the hospital environment.

Perhaps drug companies could research how hypnotherapy affects the brain to develop better drugs. Eventually, more and more people going under hypnotherapy will allow us to understand that it is an effective approach within a whole pantheon of treatment options. There are hundreds of thousands of hypnotherapists globally and many of them are developing their approaches and these can be pulled together, researched, and understood.

I came into hypnotherapy a long time ago and during my student years, you didn't connect depression and hypnotherapy. People like Michael[8] Yapko were researching and understanding that hypnotherapy has a significant role to play in treating depression and now it has become one of the recommended approaches to treat depression, especially in conjunction with CBT. There were lots of controversies, and it is about studying and finding out. I.e. there is still controversy about treating epilepsy with hypnotherapy. But new research is showing that seizures can be managed with hypnotherapy. Research has shown that hypnotherapy can help to manage diabetes and a specific lifestyle.

We need to get ourselves out there and do positive things to help get rid of the misconceptions. I must say I am hearing fewer misconceptions when I tell people I am a hypnotherapist. In the early days, people would say things like "Don't look into his eyes" or "He will make you cluck like a chicken with a click of a finger" but now more and more people are expressing interest in what it can do to help. People are starting to understand the difference between hypnosis for entertainment and hypnosis for overcoming health issues.

How have results of this research been brought forward into the public sphere to bring an understanding of the mind and body connection and what positive role has hypnotherapy here?

Media- we need more media reports on it. It is somewhat out there, and anyone following hypnotherapy on social media gets promoted. It is encouraging that the media is picking up on this research; things like NICE[9], they are starting to see where hypnotherapy has recommendations of treatments, and it is recommended for IBS, pain management, pre-natal and Hypno-birth. So these recommendations have slowly started to trickle through. We as therapists can spread the news via social media, giving talks in the broadcasting media. It needs a bit more effort. Right now the interest is in Brexit and covid and, mainly covid in the UK. Once the media starts to focus on the wider range of issues again, hopefully, it will pick up some of the positive things that have been going on.

We are doing open sessions for the public in LSCCH for experiencing hypnotherapy in a safe environment. Right now it is online. This experience tells the general public about what hypnotherapy can do. I have identified from some of my group therapy that people love the hypnosis-induced relaxation aspect. It helps to understand that there is another way to deal with some of the issues they are concerned about. When therapists will be out there doing good work, it is word of the mouth that will bring an awareness of it.

In terms of the future of research in hypnotherapy, any message for the students and practitioners of clinical hypnotherapy?

There is an abundance of interesting literature out there on the subject. Read as much as you can. We know that to have access to some of these papers a fee is required. Luckily at LSCCH, we have access to a large number of papers including BSCH and there are papers available online under the creative commons license. Google Scholar will give access to research papers so search as much as you can. It is extremely important to stay informed and updated on knowledge. Who knows, many of the students and practitioners will go on to develop new techniques.

Any last message?

Hypnosis must be doing something because some of the things we call hypnosis techniques today have been practised since the dawn of history; before the invention of chemical anaesthesia, people from all over the world would go to see and learn from James Esdaile in India who was using hypnotherapy (Mesmerism as it was then called in Europe). It is robust and out there. It has always existed. It has been pushed aside for profit-related causes and it was made into an unattractive method. But it keeps coming back consistently in the medical arena. More people are training as hypnotherapists, more medics are using hypnotherapists. My message to the drug company is if you invest in the research of hypnotherapy, it will eventually bring profit to you.

The audio version of this interview in detail is available on https://ihypnosis.live

[1] The brachial plexus is the network of nerves that sends signals from the spinal cord to the shoulder, arm, and hand.

[2] Philosopher René Descartes: The theory that the mental and the physical, or mind and body or mind and brain, are, in some sense, radically different kinds of things.

[3] Cytokines are small proteins that are crucial in controlling the growth and activity of other immune system cells and blood cells.

[4] To relieve from Carpal Tunnel Syndrome; is pressure on a nerve on the wrist causing tingling, numbness and severe pain on the hand and fingers, especially at night.

[5] The somatosensory cortex is located in the parietal lobe, have numerous functions, including representation of the body, tactile attention, sensorimotor integration, and the processing of painful stimuli, empathy, and emotion.

[6] The anterior cingulate cortex, or ACC, is found at the front of the cingulate cortex and wraps around the head of the corpus callosum implicating complex cognitive functions such as empathy, impulse, control, emotions and decision making.

[7] Benzodiazepines: Group of sedative medication

[8] Michael Yapko: Internationally recognized American Psychotherapist and Hypnotherapist

[9] National Institute of Health & Care Excellence

HYPNOTHERAPY DIRECTORY

Karen Puttick
Clinical Hypnotherapist

E-mail: karen@chilternhypnotherapy.co.uk
Websites: www.karenputtick.com and www.chilternhypnotherapy.co.uk

Jason Demant
North End Road
London, NW 11 7PH
Phone: 07862 494634

Website: www.deepdivetherapy.co.uk
E-mail: info@deepdivetherapy.co.uk

Coaching with NLP

Phone: 07947 099280
UK Freephone: 08000835797

Website: https://www.coachingwithnlp.co/
E-mail: wayne@coachingwithnlp.co
Twitter: https://twitter.com/wayne_farrell
Facebook: https://www.facebook.com/CoachingWithNLP

Christopher Wadsworth
Board Certified Coach, Clinical Hypnotherapist
Geneva, Switzerland
Tel. +41 (0)22 508 7509
https://authenticlifecoaching.ch/
https://swisshypnotherapy.ch/
chris@authenticlifecoaching.ch

Stephen Travers, Advanced Hypnotherapy

Email: stephen@stravershypnosis.com
Website: https://stravershypnosis.com/
Facebook: https://www.facebook.com/stravershypnotherapy

Richard J D'Souza (B.A. Hons., P.G.C.E., D.C. Hyp.)

Address of the practice: The Therapy Centre, 33 The Parade, Roath, Cardiff, CF24 3AD

Telephone: 07738 938197
E-mail: info@clinicalhypnotherapy-cardiff.co.uk
Website: https://www.clinicalhypnotherapy-cardiff.co.uk
Price for the session: £70

Brian Jacobs – Hypnotic Solutions

Address of the practice: Finchley, London N3 3LF

Telephone: 02084468061
E-mail: brian@hypnoticsolutions.co.uk
Website: https://www.hypnoticsolutions.co.uk/

Jakub Tencl Ph.D. – iHypnosis®

Address of the practice: Westend Medical Practice, 6 Bendall Mews, NW1 6SN, London

Telephone: 07704 734 834
E-mail: info@ihypnosis.org.uk
Website: https://www.ihypnosis.org.uk

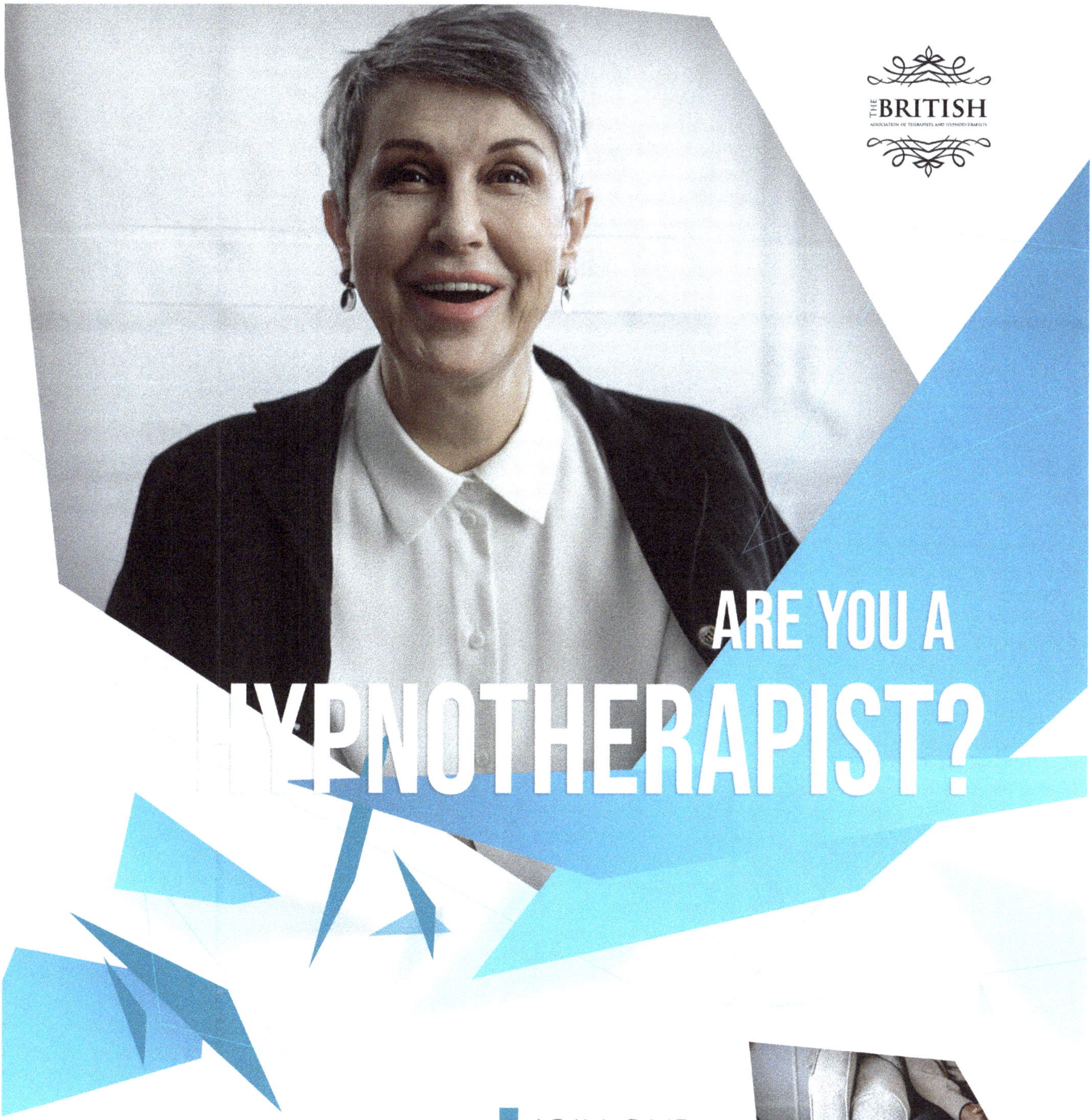

ARE YOU A HYPNOTHERAPIST?

THE BRITISH
ASSOCIATION OF THERAPISTS AND HYPNOTHERAPISTS

The British Association of Therapists and Hypnotherapists is an unincorporated association established in 2013.

| CONTACT US AT

info@britishassociationoftherapists.co.uk

| JOIN OUR ASSOCIATION

We are open to **42 disciplines** and provide attractive benefits.

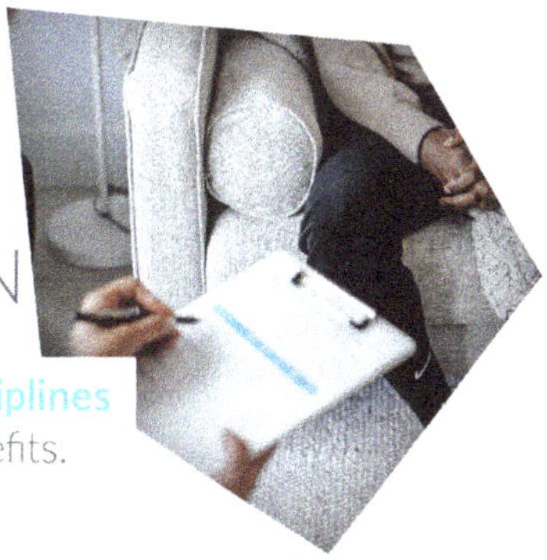

www.facebook.com/spreadinglightbat/   britishassociationoftherapists.co.uk

INTERVIEWS

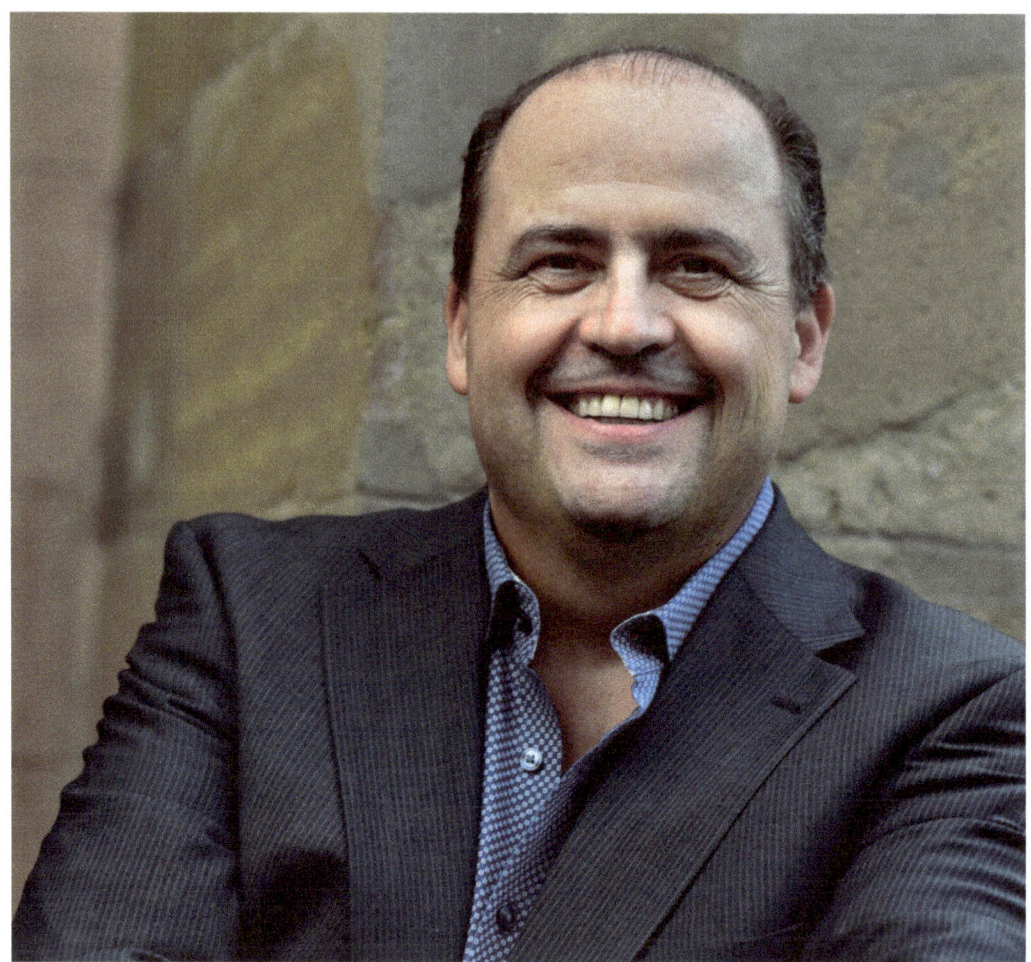

HANSRUEDI WIPF;
AN EDUCATOR OF CLINICAL HYPNOTHERAPY

Omni Hypnosis Training Centre; changing lives Worldwide

It was 1985, a young man in America watched a stage hypnosis show and came out with sparkling interest in what hypnosis truly means in modern term. He picked up a book and the journey begun of acquiring knowledge on what is hypnosis, how does it work, what is the myth behind it and why should we receive clinical hypnotherapy. The man is Hansruedi Wipf and today is the owner and the chairman of World's largest hypnotherapy school, Omni Hypnosis Centre.

> Interviews   > by: Shanta Sultana   > e: shanta.sultana@hypnosis.plus

INTERVIEWS

Omni Hypnosis is situated in Switzerland and has training centres in twenty six countries, over fifty locations in four continents. Coming up to forty two years, Omni Hypnosis was born in 1979 under Gerald Kein and has produced over fourteen thousand students who are working over eighty countries around the globe, improving lives for the better.

Omni hypnosis is the first ISO9001 certified Hypnosis Training Worldwide; ISO9001 is a globally recognised certification, meaning it is the ultimate global benchmark for quality management for an institution.

The Swiz personality Hanruedi started watching videos of the legendary hypnotist Gerald Kein in around 1998 and fascinated by the prospects of healing and helping people, Hansruedi opted for hypnosis training in Florida and became a devoted student of Kein. Trained by the master himself, Hansruedi became Kein's successor in 2012 however; Kein continued to support Omni Hypnosis until his death in 2017.

"It took me many years to study and come to this point and I am still continuing to know more", tells a very humble Hansruedi , who has brought his years of experience working in the automobile industry, in the entrepreneurial World and in the field of sports, in three countries, made Omni Hypnosis an international ground for training and researching clinical hypnotherapy.

Hansruedi, the author of Hypnosis - Health and Healing in Natural Way believes in the unity of human beings transcending all barriers and has an internal desire in helping and healing people from all walks of life. Omni Hypnosis does not drag clients to the therapy sessions for months after months; instead it offers what is needed over a limited numbers of session hence fast affective help without the stress of attending numbers of meetings and tasks.

Hanruedi uses the making of an automobile and the capacity of a racing driver as a metaphor to explain what makes a good hypnotherapist and how it works on the clients and continues to progress the standard of Omni Hypnosis whilst maintaining the philosophy of Kein. The height of this progress is the largest scientific project on hypnotherapy, research on how hypnotherapy actually works and how it affects different networks of the brain, is to be releasing in 2021, and it is the first of its kind.

Hanruedi, kindly offered his valuable time in conversation with Hypnosis Plus.

What do you think are motivational routes for studying hypnotherapy?'
Motivational routes can be very different; some people decide to study hypnotherapy after having a positive personal experience. They realise that hypnotherapy can provide them with a solution to a problem in only a few sessions. This sparks their interest, and they feel motivated to learn hypnosis themselves and perhaps help other people to solve their problems quickly and effectively. There are people who are interested in becoming hypnotherapists and others who are just curious to find out more about it.

If a paramedic and medical staff for instance want to learn an effective tool that can help people promptly, they might want to study hypnotherapy. Working in a healthcare environment, they usually live for a higher purpose and want to help people to lead a better life and possibly find their higher purpose, too.

Then there are people who simply want to experience hypnosis and find out more about it, they enjoy talking about hypnosis and sharing their learning experience with their family and friends. I would say they make up roughly twenty percent of our students.

People from all walks of life are motivated to study hypnotherapy. But I would say that a major motivational route is the profound personal experience and the realisation that hardly any other method can bring about a change in people's lives in such a short period of time.

Who can study hypnotherapy? Does it require somehow a specific personality?
I taught hypnosis to my nephews and nieces when they were about nine or ten years old. It is not difficult at all to learn how to hypnotise someone, on the contrary, it is very easy. People can learn self-hypnosis in one or one and a half hours. Nowadays, there is a vast number of schools that teach hypnosis and hypnotherapy. And basically, anyone can sign up for it. In my opinion, anyone should be able to learn the art of hypnosis and find out how this might change their lives. To study hypnotherapy, however, it helps to be mature to handle the more challenging issues in life, to have intuition and empathy – and a big portion of life experience.

Why would someone want to study hypnotherapy?
As mentioned earlier, people might want to study hypnotherapy because they want to be able to help others quickly and effectively. Studying hypnotherapy at our training centre, for instance, students will acquire a reproducible, easy to learn and apply hypnosis method that is ISO 9001 certified and has a high success rate. We have doctors, naturopathic practitioner, and psychotherapists or people who seek a change in their careers who study hypnotherapy. But you do not have to have a medical or psychological background to help people. You might feel that it is time for you to reach out to your higher purpose, to help people and do something for the higher good. If you want to work with minds and emotions to foster mental health, hypnotherapy is what you want to study.

Is there any ethical issue that is, in particular, to be concerned in terms of the field of study of hypnotherapy and what should the potential students and the existing students be aware of?
I am not worried about ethical issues. A lot of people have a misconception of hypnosis because they might have seen a stage show, they might be worried to go into hypnosis and lose control or become manipulated. Hypnotherapy is a whole different story. Hypnotherapy helps people to solve problems and allows them to get back the control of their lives that they might have lost in the course of stressful events, pain or illness. In our training centre, we follow strict ethical guidelines and all of our instructors sign a business code of conduct. This sets very high standards on how they deliver their lessons, how they interact with their students, and how they teach ethical compliance. Students will learn how to handle their clients' confidential information, but also how not to prolong sessions for financial benefits if the clients' problems can be solved quickly. For example, if a car has broken breaks, the mechanic shouldn't keep fixing one break at a time and asking the car owner to return; instead, the mechanic should fix all four breaks at once. This means that we do not break down the process into more sessions than is required and keep

INTERVIEWS

asking the clients to come back. Financial gain should never be the motivation for becoming a hypnotherapist. Instead, there must be an inherent desire to help people. A good income will eventually be the result of good therapy and happy clients.

There are hypnotists who take interest in a different thought direction; few of them are based on the theories from the earlier centuries. In your opinion, does it cause confusion in the public understanding of what really hypnosis is and is this an obstacle for the hypnotherapists who want to practice hypnotherapy clinically?
If you look at the history of any business, you will see that they have faced a lot of challenges and perhaps made wrong decisions to come up to a set standard and understanding. For example, there was a time when they used to put cocaine in cola, or when smoking was recommended by doctors. But we have learnt and improved over time and we don't do those things anymore. This is how a profession develops. People have to try and practice things to understand what works and what doesn't. That is a normal evolutionary process of any profession.

As for public understanding: what causes confusion and what doesn't? Let's say stage hypnosis causes confusion. Actually, stage hypnotists are very good at entertaining. And part of the legacy of stage hypnotism is that we have learnt something about it from them. Stage hypnotists work under a lot of pressure to offer a show people are willing to pay for. I personally don't have any problem with stage hypnosis. I see it more as a problem of general education about how stage hypnosis works and what hypnosis is and what it is not. There are thousands of hypnotherapists and practitioners out there helping people to change or solve their problems. If we educate people to better understand hypnosis and hypnotherapy, then both can coexist for their own reasons.

There are fear and doubt about hypnotherapy from the perspective of communities that are associating hypnosis with unsolicited and supernatural intervention. In your opinion, how these thoughts came up and how can they be overcome?
There are numerous communities who cherish their own theories and have their own opinions about hypnosis, calling it a deviant practice or suggesting it puts a spell on people. I don't worry about them at all. We can try to educate people, but if they want to cling to their particular beliefs, we cannot change their minds. It is our task to judge religious delusion. I rather focus on those who show a sincere interest in our work.

Is there any particular ethical issue in the field of hypnotherapy practice you are concerned about? What can be done about this?
As mentioned earlier, we have a solid business code of conduct; this is why I do not worry about ethical issues in our trainings. We use a method called "Regression to cause and fix it". This means that we tackle the cause of the client's problem and do not focus on symptoms. You probably have heard of Dave Elman, the noted American Hypnotist who came up with easy and quick hypnosis techniques that can solve a problem within one session. The founder of OMNI Hypnosis Gerald F. Kein was Elman's student and he kept Elman's techniques alive through OMNI. Kein improved and refined Elman's methods so they can be taught, easily learnt, and applied. Helping clients as fast as possible is in my opinion the most ethical thing to do. So it is not the ethical issues in the clinical hypnotherapy I am worried about, but the many misconceptions that may make people think that there are ethical issues.

You have a hypnotherapy school all around the globe. Do you take a different approach in teaching based on the locations or do you have a set of specific rules of ethics?
It doesn't matter at what corner of the earth the clients are, what unites all of us humans are our basic feelings in relation to pain, love, happiness and so on. This is why we have training centres in Europe, Asia, Africa, and South America and know that the training is the same in all locations. The business code of conduct is exactly the same in every school around the globe, so is the training curriculum. We guarantee trained instructors and a specific standard of teaching. It means I should be able to turn up in any class situated in any part of the World on day five, six, or seven and I should be hearing exactly the same thing. What is taught in all OMNI schools is the same, so I shouldn't have to spend time worrying about what the students are learning. When Kein established the school in 1979, he created the standard maintaining the teaching of Elman. Elman's method of Regression to cause became OMNI's technique and Kein became our legacy. We still use Regression to cause, and much more: We teach Universal Therapy, Ultra Height® and Ultra Healing®, and much more. Usually, with no more than one to three sessions, eighty percent of all problems are resolved. We have numerous video recordings proving such successes. In the end, our utmost concern at every school is respect towards other human beings. It is of fundamental importance to gain the trust of our clients – no matter where in the World they are. The success of our students is our success. And our students change lives.

Omni Hypnosis arranges annual Hypnosis Convention in Zurich every autumn, involving over forty speakers and fifty presentations, an essential gathering for the learners and practitioners who are cordially invited from across the globe.

Hansruedi informs, continuing to collect clients' experience and cases being videotaped as proofs of affective hypnotherapy are a part of the ongoing educational strategy to understand modern hypnotherapy. "No other profession can do what we can do; it is possible to solve a problem in two or three sessions" Hansruedi extends the importance of educating the public about hypnotherapy and advocates Hypnosis Plus continuing to work on it.

To find out how hypnotherapy can help you go to https://hypnosis.plus/

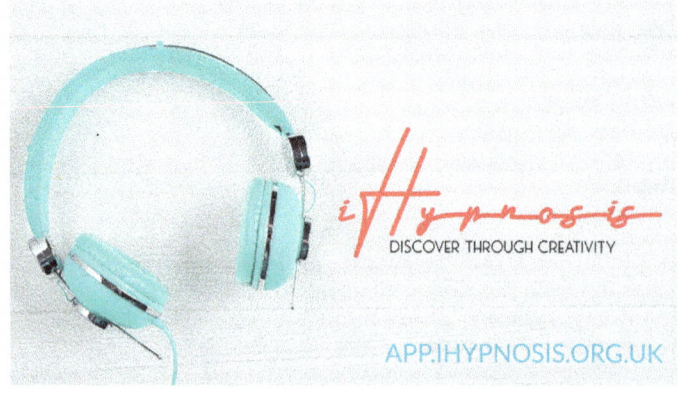

iHypnosis
DISCOVER THROUGH CREATIVITY

APP.IHYPNOSIS.ORG.UK

Is there a life after the Pandemic?
A positive afternoon with Wayne Farrell

How can a solution-focused mind free us from anxiety and fear?

"Tell me, what is your biggest fear in the pandemic?"

I talk about work security, monetary stability, uncertain career prospects, and how it may be months down the line.

"Close your eyes for a bit." Well, how was I supposed to disobey the instruction from the life coach and the hypnotherapist who is improving lives globally? Using Neuro-Linguistic Programming (NLP), Liverpool-based South African Life Coach, Wayne Farrell, continues to assist people from all over the world with fear, anxiety, depression, and stress. Coming up to twenty-three years in the UK, Wayne has travelled wide and plans to take his work as far as Central America.

"Let's take a timeline from now up to Christmas 2021," Wayne told me as my eyes were now closed. He asked me to use my imagination. "Imagine step by step, all the things you would like to achieve, they are happening, and by Christmas, you have achieved all the things you have. Keep picturing, keep picturing things that you want, you have them, one at a time". Was it the power of speech or my willingness to submit to such imagination? I found myself smiling whilst my eyes were closed. I felt warmth and a sense of excitement, feeling "what if!"

"You can open your eyes now." So I did. I was now grinning.

"So, how does it feel?" Asked Wayne beaming with a smile.

"Very good," I said honestly.

"Well, that wasn't so hard, was it?"

No, it wasn't, I thought, and I realised I felt happy as well. It didn't feel like short-term happiness.

So is it that easy? Can we actually work on our anxiety and fear during the pandemic with the power of our imagination and thoughts? Cynics might say it actually has no meaning in the context of reality. The reality is, we don't have many opportunities at the end of this pandemic to re-build ourselves. It is because people are trying to believe in it and submitting to it to be influenced by such thoughts. "It is what we feed our mind and what we feed our body," Said Wayne. Well, that makes sense, doesn't it? Our good health depends on what we eat, and without good health, we cannot perform the desired tasks. Therefore, if we don't feed our minds with the right kind of thoughts, we may not find alleyways and alternative roots to get where we want to get in our career and personal lives.

Confronting adverse situations and many hardships as a child, Wayne wanted to be a better dad and a positive example for his son. So he went for a life coaching course and saw what amazing changes could be possible with the power of thoughts and the positive changes in our world views. Wayne then completed NLP Practitioner Training and felt that he has more to give than just giving himself the power of positivity. He started educating people in various parts of the world with life coaching, hypnotherapy, business coaching, and mindfulness, to state the few. Wayne plans to create a sustainable farm in Panama where he will offer these services as well as donate the production of the farm to children in need and to people who are suffering from difficult situations.

INTERVIEWS

"First the basic," Says Wayne, "Food for the body to be strong and then food for the mind for how to build a future. I don't believe only a few people should have the right to have economic stability, I believe everyone has the right to economic comfort, and everyone has the right to believe they can have it with the right kind of tools. I believe it is possible. So the training comes later, once their basic needs are fulfilled." Wayne explains, "But I shall continue to help my clients all over the world as well."

So how can we not be afraid during the pandemic about our future? Hypnosis Plus had the pleasure to interview Wayne Farrell and had the opportunity to do a crash course on how to change the way we think.

What is anxiety? How may we identify anxiety, and what means a disorder in the frame of anxiety?

The term - disorder, I don't really buy it. The problem in life is we have these labels. Disorder is a label on someone. When I have a disorder, I am a victim. I am not a believer in labelling people with terms such as disorder because it victimises people, and it is difficult to receive help once you are a victim.

Anxiety is fear - fear of something happening or not happening. For example, people may think covid will start a great depression in the economy, and they then become scared. They start imagining what will happen to them, what will happen to their family, that people will die, and everything that they are scared of. Anxiety is the fear of a badly constituted future. When you picture the bad thing, you are anxious about it.

How could anxiety disorder develop? What is the difference between natural anxiety and disorder in the same frame? Do we develop it gradually, or does it hit us at once?

To start with, lots of people turn to medicines such as anti-depressants.

Now let's look at this.

For example, my daughter was anxious about her SATS exam some time ago. It is not a bad thing. It means she wanted to do well. So she needed to imagine that she will do well. In these circumstances, if you think, let's imagine it will go well, you will do well. Another example is, if I want this interview to be well, then I shall think about it, it means I want it to do well. So a little anxiousness in life is needed to do well or to achieve something as long as it does not go out of control. So it is when we lose control of our thoughts and imagination, it is about having control over our thoughts.

Let me use another example; a husband comes home for dinner at 6 o'clock. It is 7 o'clock today, but he isn't here. He is not answering the phone, and the wife starts to imagine all the negatives, such as he had an accident, is seeing someone else, etc. She is losing control over her thoughts, and anxiety will hit her. So we have to look at the root of the cause of the anxiety. Doctors work on the symptomology of a patient; hence the patient gets medication or anti-depressant to control the anxiety. Symptomology is a set of symptoms of a medical condition shown in a patient, but that doesn't solve the route of the problem. If we work with the root cause of those anxious thoughts, anxiety diminishes. Depression doesn't have a place if we deal with fear. So going back to the wife, she needs to find out why she had jumped to a negative conclusion.

To understand the root of the cause and the remedy based on Symptomology, let's imagine I am hitting my head constantly. Eventually, I shall have a headache, and if I go to the doctor, he will give me medication to control the headache because I have shown the symptoms of having a headache. But this will not solve the problem because I shall hit my head again, and the headaches will be recurring. So I shall always be in those medications. But if someone works on the root of the problem, that is, I am hitting my head and try to find out why my behaviour is this way, then at some point, I

INTERVIEWS

shall stop that behaviour; so I shall not have a headache again, and I won't need the medication anymore.

So we need to find out the root cause of the problem, and once we have found out why we are behaving in a certain way or thinking in a certain way, it will be possible to be free from anxiety and depression.

Tell us, once we are identifying anxiety issues, what can we do? What can we do as friends or family for the person who is suffering from anxiety, especially during the pandemic? Please give us an example.

We need to have control over the way we think. Remember that it is what we feed our mind and what we feed our body? We need to allow us to find the root cause of the anxiety and change the way we have been thinking.

As family and friends, we can really support the person who is suffering. We need to make them feel safe, feel loved, and show them that they are not alone.

What are the must-not and must when we suffer from anxiety?

We need to stop looking for evidence for things to go wrong. Stop overthinking. Stop thinking that things will go wrong. Take control over your thoughts and change the way you are seeing things, seeing the future. So to change the way you think, you need to look at **TOP**.

T: **Take** control over your thoughts and take control to change them.

O: Think, what are my **Options**? What other outcome could come out of this situation? How can I get the outcome to be true? Perhaps I could study, read more, do online courses, and take control of my health.

P: **Practice** focusing on what you want instead. When you are catching yourself imagining things going wrong, stop. Think again, what your options are, and start practicing focusing on what you want.

Michel de Montaigne, the French philosopher, said, "My life has been full of terrible misfortunes, most of which never happened."

What it means that we imagine about things that will go wrong for no purpose. We must not keep thinking about what may go wrong; it brings doom and gloom, and it leads to losing life's purpose, and when we don't see the results, we believe we are right about imagining what could have gone wrong. I work with my clients about what they are feeling, what makes them imagine how things will go wrong, and work on how to stop that way of thinking. But everyone is different, and there is no single answer. You cannot just do one standard thing with all the clients because there isn't a single answer for all the clients. I work with each client, and there are different approaches you need to have rather than using a single technique because everyone is different.

Are we able to allocate most of the time we have during the pandemic for working on mental health? How?

Of course, there is the opportunity with the time we have in the pandemic. Mental health includes so much; it is a big question. Think about what the mental health issues are that we are dealing with and what help we can get. There is psychotherapy, hypnotherapy, alternative therapy, educating ourselves, and find out what actually is the root of the problem. Always go back to what I told you about what you feed your body and what you feed your mind. Think; when we exercise, our body releases a chemical called endorphin, which triggers a positive feeling. We feel better and healthier. We are not going to feel the same way if we are less physically active. So the same way, if we don't keep our minds active and engage in self-improvements, we won't have much to look forward to. We have to keep running that hamster wheel.

The negative aspect of the pandemic is the lack

INTERVIEWS

of opportunities because of redundancies, economic issues, and restrictions on the face to face communications. It seems reasonable to state that it is not possible to make the best use of our time because the prospects of re-building ourselves seem bleak. Tell us how we can work around these issues that are currently affecting us.

Easy answer; well, it seems easy, that is, create your own reality. Create your own economic situation. It seems easy to say, I know, but it is also possible in reality. There are ways we can do things, and we can change things around. For example, my business has changed dramatically in the last twelve months. I have always helped people face to face, but I had to think of other ways in the pandemic. I now help clients online. You have to look for opportunities within the situation of reality, and there are things you will be able to think of. For example, you know Sir Isaac Newton, the great mathematician and physicist of Cambridge University, right? In 1665, the great plague broke out, and all the students were sent home. For twelve months, there were no classes, everything was closed, so it was like the lockdown today. Rather than visualising a negative future, Newton used the time in isolation to solve the most unsolvable mathematical problem. He spent two years in the pandemic developing his theories in gravity, calculus, and the law of motion. It means he focused on himself during the lockdown and what could he do with the time available in the pandemic. Sure, one may say, but he was a genius! But remember that he didn't start out as a genius. That first twelve months were a great opportunity to think about his theories, and he did it without any help of the professors in the pandemic when there was total isolation. Take it as an example, you don't start out as something, but you need to develop on it. You can use this time to help your children to develop something, think about what you can do with them that could be good for their wellbeing. You could learn something together, read, make something, and ask them about ideas. Unfortunately, we have been spending most of our time on Netflix, but there is more you can do with the time you have been offered so that at the end of the pandemic, you have something. And that is what you can take from Newton's example.

What advice do you have for the people who are naturally worried about the future or the safety of the vaccines and working environments?

Jim Rohn, the American entrepreneur, author, and a motivator, said, "For things to change, you have to change."

If I want things to be changed, I need to do things differently. Think about an example of you wanting to lose weight. To lose the weight, you have to make the changes in your habits and lifestyle that is conducive to your expectation. If you want to have change, you need to make changes; in fact, change is the only constant. There are always changes. You need to change something inside.

"If the rate of change on the outside exceeds the rate of change on the inside, the end is near" - Jack Welsh.

Yes, it is an alienating experience in the pandemic, a total change in our experience. Imagine somebody has time travelled from the 16th century. How would they feel? How shocking our lives would seem to them? They would be physically here, but internally, they would be in the sixteenth century. They have not made that internal change. So the pandemic may feel that way, but we humans have to constantly evolve. We need to learn how to adopt, we need to accept that changes are constant, and we need to adapt to changes. A good example is the successful business people who constantly have to change according to the changes around them.

We have been made redundant. So think how we can evolve from this point. What are my interests? What other skill sets do I have that I can make use of? How can we be invaluable to

INTERVIEWS

an organisation?

For example, my wife is a Teaching Assistant. Unfortunately, there were redundancies in her institution, twice. Nevertheless, she kept her job. So I now ask her to think about what else she can think about to make herself invaluable to the organisation or what other things she could do to move further and up.

Remember that each person is different. We have our own values and beliefs. If I start criticising your faith and values, we shall end up in conflict. We have deeply seated believes, which makes us indifferent to changes. But we cannot start criticising everyone for their beliefs.

What you have to do is think about the things like pro-vaccine and anti-vaccine theories. It is good that we can question things, and we can suspect things. But it boils down to facts, not theories based on a belief system. Don't start believing everything you read on the internet or the videos on YouTube. Try to understand the facts around these videos and news on social networks.

Think about the changes you need to make at the moment from the social point of view and adapt to those changes. For example, personally, I don't believe the mask doesn't affect the students' learning ability. The pupils are sitting there with their mouth covered, they can't have that full face to face contact with tutors, they are sitting there breathing the same air, it is uncomfortable and unclean, i.e., they could sneeze inside the mask, and they have to sit on it all day. But from the societal point of view, they need to follow the protocol.

So you have to think about what I can do to have better control in me and have better control in my environment. People don't have control if people are not adapted to change. So do things from the social point of view and try not to believe in theories that are not fact-based.

Do you have some motivational words for the time after the pandemic?

There are few things you need to look at.

Focus on what you want and what outcome you want.
What would you have done if you knew that you would fail?
How do you absolutely know that you would fail?
Is it absolutely true that you would fail?
What would happen if you tried and actually achieved it?
When do you start?

When you keep picturing the failure, you will be anxious, and you will stop trying something different. It doesn't mean you will fail. You need to change from being a problem-focused person to a solution-focused person. A solution-focused mind will change the focus externally. Remember about what we feed our mind.

Picturing a problem-focused future can be installed in us. For example, a child can pick up a negative message from the parents' negative outlook and grow up with a negative focus in life. To understand it, think about a baby elephant. It is tied up as a baby, and it knows it cannot go further. When it's unchained as an adult elephant, it still walks around the same loop because as a baby, it learned that it could only move around in a particular area. So it never thinks of running away. We feel we can't do something, and we are unable to succeed because we are also circling the same loop of thoughts.

The thing is, when you think negatively, everything will turn out to be negative because you have not cut off that chain that trained you to stay in the same place.

But a solution-focused mind can be achieved. Stop focusing on the doom and gloom and start thinking about things like how I can create my own economy. It can be self-taught, so when will you start?

www.ingramcontent.com/pod-product-compliance
Lightning Source LLC
Chambersburg PA
CBHW050145180526
45172CB00011B/1319